HISTORY

ARTS FOR HEALTH

Series Editor: Paul Crawford, Professor of Health Humanities, University of Nottingham, UK

The *Arts for Health* series offers a ground-breaking set of books that guide the general public, carers and healthcare providers on how different arts can help people to stay healthy or improve their health and wellbeing.

Bringing together new information and resources underpinning the health humanities (that link health and social care disciplines with the arts and humanities), the books demonstrate the ways in which the arts offer people worldwide a kind of shadow health service – a non-clinical way to maintain or improve our health and wellbeing. The books are aimed at general readers along with interested arts practitioners seeking to explore the health benefits of their work, health and social care providers and clinicians wishing to learn about the application of the arts for health, educators in arts, health and social care and organisations, carers and individuals engaged in public health or generating healthier environments. These easy-to-read, engaging short books help readers to understand the evidence about the value of arts for health and offer guidelines, case studies and resources to make use of these non-clinical routes to a better life.

Other Titles in the Series:

Magic	Richard Wiseman
Video	John Quin
Body Art	Brian Brown and Virginia Kuulei Berndt

Forthcoming Titles

Games	Sandra Danilovic
Creative Writing	Mark Pearson and Helen Foster
Dancing	Noyale Colin and Kathryn Stamp

HISTORY

BY

ANNA GREENWOOD
University of Nottingham, UK

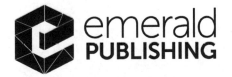

United Kingdom – North America – Japan – India
Malaysia – China

Emerald Publishing Limited
Emerald Publishing, Floor 5, Northspring, 21-23 Wellington Street,
Leeds LS1 4DL.

First edition 2023

British Library Cataloguing in Publication Data
A catalogue record for this book is available from the British Library

ISBN: 978-1-80455-188-2 (Print)
ISBN: 978-1-80455-185-1 (Online)
ISBN: 978-1-80455-187-5 (Epub)

INVESTOR IN PEOPLE

For Hanni and David

CONTENTS

ABOUT THE AUTHOR

Anna Greenwood is Professor of Health History at the University of Nottingham, UK. She is the author of several books and articles examining various aspects of modern health history, focussing on social and cultural dimensions. Her works include examinations of western medicine under British colonial rule, the dissemination of British retail pharmacy along global pathways, the history of Florence Nightingale, and the history of addictive products in the sponsorship of modern professional sport. She is an advocate for the health humanities and is co-editor of a series for *Intellect Books: The Global Health Humanities.*

ABOUT THE CASE
STUDY AUTHORS

Andres S. Dobat works at Aarhus University in Denmark as an Associate Professor doing research and projects which make archaeology and heritage relevant for all – be it as a building stone for inclusive and democratic societies or to mitigate mental health challenges.

Geoffery Z. Kohe is Senior Lecturer in Sport Management and Policy in the School of Sport and Exercise Sciences, University of Kent. He has interdisciplinary research expertise in global, transnational and local sport and physical activity landscapes, with specific emphasis on organisational politics and capacity building, stakeholder network formations and national and international governing body relationships.

Coreen McGuire is Lecturer in Twentieth-Century British History at Durham University. Her first book *Measuring Difference, Numbering Normal* showed how the data sets used in interwar audiometry and spirometry impacted disability definition. She was recently awarded a 5-year Wellcome University Award for her project, 'When Categories Constrain Care: Investigating Social Categories in Health Norms Through Disability History 1909–1958'.

Chris Russell works at the Association for Dementia Studies, at the University of Worcester, UK, as a Senior Lecturer. He is the author of several articles on dementia, citizenship, leisure and physical activity. He is currently Co-editor of a new book, *Leisure and Everyday Life with Dementia*, to be published by Open University Press in Autumn 2023.

Aja Smith, Ph.D. Anthropology, is a   post-doctorate in Andres Dobat's *Vetektor Buddy Program*, Aarhus University. Her research has revolved around professional training, personal development, self-therapy, contemporary spirituality, multispecies anthropology and methodology, and has mainly been based in Denmark. Her work is published in *Ethos*, *Medical Anthropology* and the creative writing outlet *Antrostorier*.

FOREWORD: CREATIVE PUBLIC HEALTH

The *Arts for Health* series aims to provide key information on how different arts and humanities practices can support, or even transform, health and wellbeing. Each book introduces a particular creative activity or resource and outlines its place and value in society, the evidence for its use in advancing health and wellbeing and cases of how this works. In addition, each book provides useful links and suggestions to readers for following-up on these quick reads. We can think of this series as a kind of shadow health service – encouraging the use of the arts and humanities alongside all the other resources on offer to keep us fit and well.

Creative practices in the arts and humanities offer a fantastic, non-medical, but medically relevant way to improve the health and wellbeing of individuals, families and communities. Intuitively, we know just how important creative activities are in maintaining or recovering our best possible lives. For example, imagine that we woke up tomorrow to find that all music, books or films had to be destroyed, learn that singing, dancing or theatre had been outlawed or that galleries, museums and theatres had to close permanently; or, indeed, that every street had posters warning citizens of severe punishment for taking photographs, drawing or writing. How would we feel? What would happen to our bodies and minds? How would we survive? Unfortunately, we have seen this kind of removal of creative activities from human society before and today many people remain terribly restricted in artistic expression and consumption.

I hope that this series adds a practical resource to the public. I hope people buy these little books as gifts for family and friends, or for hard-pressed healthcare professionals, to encourage them to revisit or to consider a creative path to living well. I hope that creative public health makes for a brighter future.

Professor Paul Crawford

ACKNOWLEDGEMENTS

Growing up as the daughter of a research scientist and a yoga teacher, I was caught between two world views. One was rational, delineated by rules, striving for cure and betterment through a dedication to learning, scientific experimentation and observation, and one was more fluid, reaching towards health and wellbeing through an ongoing journey of mind, body and spirit expansion. While my father worked in a laboratory and lectured to halls full of medical students, my mother brought equilibrium and companionship to members of our community, as she guided them through their sun salutes in the local church halls. In our suburban semidetached house, allopathic medicine and a holistic view of health co-existed under one roof.

It seems quite fitting that I am now a Professor of Health History. Historians need rigour, discipline, imagination and creativity in equal measure. While history relies on evidence, it is nothing without interpretation. What is less discussed is that history can also provide us with new avenues and toolkits to think about and experience the world. These insights and techniques, furthermore, can improve health and wellbeing. They can do this at the personal, communal and structural levels, both mentally and physically.

This modest contribution to the Emerald *Arts for Health* series probes the role that reading, writing, advocating with and participating in history can play in extending health and wellbeing. I am very conscious that it represents a start rather than a definitive guide and I take full responsibility for any faults, omissions or oversights. It is a work which sits on the shoulders of many excellent researchers. While it has been a joy reading so many various insightful contributions to the subfield, this book can claim to be no more than an accessible introduction, signposting areas where people can look to access more in-depth analyses.

My thanks are particularly extended to the case study authors who are presented within this book. Andres Dobat, Geoffery Kohe, Coreen McGuire, Chris Russell and Aja Smith: I am really thankful for your insightful contributions and for allowing me to showcase your research in this way. I also extend my warm thanks to Paul Crawford, who as well as being a source of constant encouragement, has taught me the benefits of thinking outside of the box. Additional thanks go to the publishing team at Emerald and the two anonymous reviewers who fed back on the proposal and improved the book's content through their shrewd recommendations. Thanks also to the Humanities Research Centre at the Australian National University in Canberra, Australia. I was privileged to take part in its Visiting Fellowship programme which, as well as introducing me to some wonderful Health Humanities scholars, provided me with some much-needed time to write up this work. It also allowed me to test some of the ideas within a seminar format and engage with enlivening discussions and feedback. Last, but by no means least, I am extremely grateful to Lisa Clarkson, whose eagle-eyed copy editing – executed with such grace and good humour – has been an immeasurable help.

I am in no doubt that this small volume is not as eloquently expressed as what my wordsmith father would have achieved. Nor is it as insightful and generously crafted as anything my mother would have guided. Nevertheless, this book curiously reflects my parents' composite influences and – because of that – it is symbolically offered as a token of my enduring love for them: Hanni (1932–2012) and David (1935–2015).

1

WHY HISTORY? AND WHY HISTORY FOR HEALTH?

We are historical animals. Both deliberatively and subconsciously, we look back over our shoulders and reach to history to situate ourselves. History helps us to understand our own life stories or the stories of those we love. History is also mobilised when we seek the stories of those we have never met, but are intrigued by, or admire. In a more disquieting vein, history reveals to us the motivations and circumstances of those who make us recoil in disbelief. History helps us to understand national and international dynamics. It allows us to make sense of the ways that political, social and economic institutions, systems and attitudes come to dominate and, sometimes, how they fall.

Needless to say, this can be an emotionally loaded process. History, when accessed in its most scholarly incarnations by analysing texts and sifting through documents in archives, can be reassuring and confirming, but it can also – in equal measure – be revelatory, ground-breaking and even shocking. Furthermore, beyond the ivory towers of formal scholarship, the discipline also works at micro- and meso-levels as a means for emotional retrieval. For example, perhaps without defining the process as historical, we engage with history when grandfather's war medals are passed around at a family reunion, when an old love letter found stuffed at the back of a drawer is shared with a new generation, when community members attend a local history talk, or when former classmates are brought back together after several years apart. As famously portrayed by Marcel Proust, deeply buried personal histories can be unlocked through re-experiencing a long-forgotten, yet fleetingly familiar, taste. For Proust, it was a madeleine momentarily dipped in a cup of lime blossom tisane. On a much more prosaic level, to this day, I cannot smell a certain brand of suntan lotion without being instantly transported back to my 10-year-old self in Germany, in the early 1980s, having the lotion liberally applied by my mother as we sat on deckchairs by a lake. Smelling that perfume never fails to reignite in my own history bank the joyful surety of being young, without responsibilities, safe and loved, while it simultaneously dredges up the buried pains of the lessons of independent adulthood, and the gnawing ache of grief in the momentary reflection that both my parents have passed.

The emotionally charged nature of engagement with history intimately links it with issues of health and wellbeing. Yet, surprisingly, history has rarely been examined in the round as a force to nourish positive health outcomes. Distinguished bodies of work have looked at the role of museums and galleries in the support of personal and public health objectives, and the role of history in health policy development – and some of those ideas are enfolded within this introductory book – but no previous work has brought together in one volume a multiplicity of approaches, viewing history centrally as a flexible and capacious tool with many health applications. History as a therapeutic agent can be accessed through interaction with objects and artefacts in community spaces of museums and galleries. It can also be mobilised through reading, writing and *doing* historical research, whether as a subject-participant or as an author. For example, history as a force for improved mental health can be demonstrated in the empathy that it evokes and the social healing it can stimulate. What is more, beyond the benefits offered through its intellectual and literary functions, history plays an important role in health policy-making by providing important precedential models or highlighting missed opportunities of the past. In several landmark legal cases involving matters of health and wellbeing, historians have played vital roles as expert witnesses, correcting assumptions that have arisen because the alternative narratives were not freely told in the past due to prevailing political, economic or social imperatives.

I am not suggesting that every therapist, carer or clinician should take a history course, nor am I denying the effectiveness of many modern western medicines or modes of health care, but I am pointing out that history runs as an invisible thread informing our connectivity to the world around us. It is in this covert, but tenacious, manner that history influences our decision-making processes about our health and our journeys to feel better or make others feel better. An awareness of this universal – albeit often hidden – evocation of earlier temporal contexts can be helpful to understand what motivates people, institutions and societies. Recognition of this elemental urge to connect with the past (or sometimes to actively disconnect from it) allows us to integrate history purposefully and carefully into our caring practices and to better understand our needs when we feel unwell or are unable to cope.

As we start this exploration, it is important first to define our parameters. What exactly do we mean when we talk about history? Who can be a historian? Where can we find history? And is it a reasonable assumption that its usefulness to modern society today can be (or should be) quarried and quantified? Finally, why might historians and health practitioners work so well together?

WHAT IS HISTORY?

At its simplest, history is the study of the past, and the historian is the interrogator of the past who aims not only to understand events and people in their own rights, but also to map and explain the complex paths of circumstances that have led to the present. As a mode of exploration which can be undertaken with scholarly precision or more casually as a hobbyist, the central investigative urge of history mirrors its original Greek etymological root, *historia*, which meant inquiry.

Even in its earliest incarnations, however, the spirit of inquiry about the past was recognised as never being entirely neutral. It was susceptible to different biases dependent on the teller. The existence of different versions or stories has long been central to the conception of the past. In Greek mythology, Clio – one of the nine muses – was upheld as the patron of history. Her job was to guide and inspire mortals to be responsible scholars and not to forget the stories from which they evolved. Herodotus, the so-called ancient Greek 'father' of history, whose nine-volume anthology *The Histories* was published in the fifth century bc, understood the importance of writing history in a way that was both engaging and securely grounded in facts. In short, Herodotus had a knack for storytelling, but he also recognised that others might have competing stories to tell, and to this end, he highlighted the importance of questioning sources and interpretations.

Storytelling as the core element of *history* can be traced through the word's journey into Middle English via France. When it first arrived in England in the late fourteenth century, as a version of the French word *estoire*, no linguistic differentiation from *story* was initially made in the English language. It took until the end of the fifteenth century for the word *history* to differentiate itself from fictional storytelling and to become associated specifically with a kind of storytelling about the past which should present a view of what *actually happened* – if possible, by citing some sort of proof.

However, although early historians used evidence and cited it to give their stories authority, it was not until the nineteenth century that this was routinely stressed as an absolutely essential requirement. It was Leopold von Ranke (1795–1886), a German historian, who led this charge and in the process has established himself as the founding father of modern professionalised history. Ranke emphasised the necessity of a sound evidential base for good history, ultimately implying that any historical subject could be studied scientifically, free from subjective bias, so long as evidence was available.

Ranke did much to ensure that the scholarly history we respect today is built on empirical data. However, the swing Ranke advocated to bring history to the lofty position of a discipline capable of being entirely neutral and always scientifically verifiable seems reductionist and simplistic to us these days. All professional historians now agree on the need for evidence, but as was argued by Herbert Butterfield in his seminal *The Whig Interpretation of History* (1931), they also accept that the writing of history is often (usually) coloured by presentist values; sometimes purposefully, sometimes unwittingly. This means that, even if historians actively try to mitigate against it, a certain degree of subjectivity comes into all historical judgements, not least those stemming from the pen of the historian as the author. It is a thorny, perhaps even impossible, challenge for even the most hyper-vigilant historian to judge events entirely on their own terms and to avoid judgements based on today's standards (Butterfield, 1931).[1] The way historians' work is coloured by our preoccupations as individuals and members of society need not be a problem. In fact, I would argue that recognising subjectivity as inherent and unavoidable is part of the intellectual fun embedded in the work of the puzzle-solving historiographer. Furthermore, conceding those bias-free interpretations of the past are impossible points to another avenue via which to study history. Ergo, historical accounts, essays, books and oral testimony become important sites of evidence for analysis in and of themselves. They are not just informative because of the facts they contain, but they are windows into the historical attitudes and preoccupations of the historians who wrote them.

From history's earliest etymological links to inquiry and storytelling to modern debates about the inevitability of subjective bias, the central tension of history can be seen, but so can some of its potentialities. It is a discipline fundamentally tied to a quest to uncover truth (even if my truth isn't necessarily your truth) through the collection and interpretation of evidence and, as such, it can ground people and reassure them. Yet, history also acknowledges, and sometimes celebrates, its capabilities as a narrative and creative practice which can entertain, mythologise, manipulate or even erase.

WHO CAN BE A HISTORIAN?

Historians can be professionals educated to apply historical methods in scholarly pursuit, or students studying in schools, colleges or universities which are enfolded in the pedagogy offered by these professionals. However, historians can also be self-taught or self-directed, working within the amateur sphere. Bearing this in mind, there tends to be differentiation – and certainly, this is so within the scholarship – between history as pursued in the academic domain and history done by 'the rest'. The latter category is usually grouped in the literature under the umbrella heading of public history.

Public history is a broad category which captures history consumed by the public, such as through popular history books and films and as displayed within museums, galleries and other public spaces. Public history also refers to the pursuit of history by members of the public actively researching history themselves. This could involve going to an archive or a library, but also might happen in private or domestic settings where individuals seek out and contextualise family artefacts or their stories. The findings from these personal investigations may well be recorded in some way (for example, in a family memoir or photo album), but they might also be experienced momentarily and retained without formal record as social memory within personal or familial contexts (Rosenzweig & Thelen, 2012).[2]

At times, the objectives of scholarly and public history can be seen to clash. One of the major pitfalls of social memory, for example, is that it can be selectively deployed to justify the teller's presentist preoccupations, or to politically mobilise groups such as those who have long endured historical invisibility. For example, a feminist might be more inclined to see feminist activism within the historical archive. For sure, oftentimes these histories can be innovatively uncovered, but sometimes, they might seem an interpretative stretch. Such an approach can sit uncomfortably with the professional historical objective to present an interpretation that gets things *right* and shows how situations happened, or how an individual or group of individuals actually felt or acted at the time. This tension sometimes puts scholars at odds with those who for valid reasons prefer nostalgic or massaged versions of the past that help to fulfil their social or political priorities in the present day. In short, there can be a fine line between uncovering a forgotten or systemically overlooked history and willing such a history into existence because it validates a current societal agenda.

Yet, despite the potential for social memory to be a site of discordance, and while it is neat and tidy to separate history into two major domains of activity, the boundaries between scholarly and public history are, in reality, blurred. Each realm informs the other, and their similarities and overlaps are more obvious than their differences. For example, there is much history that goes on in the non-academic domain which is carefully and meticulously analysed. Hobbyist historians often refer to scholarly published texts and frequently have become adept and enthusiastic in their sleuthing for historical evidence, as the craze for family history has demonstrated. Furthermore, since the boom in the 1960s in the study of social history, everyday experiences have been as interesting to many professional historians as seminal moments of nationally celebrated importance. Subsequently, public history has become an important branch of history, worthy of academic analysis in its own right. Historians working within this sub-discipline often cite social memories within their scholarly publications. In fact, although the academic historian should not give up on the centrality of evidence for historical narratives and reconstructions, it is recognised that one of their analytic jobs is to unpick and contextualise nostalgia and retrospective meaning-making. Studying how people create a scaffold which gives meaning to them, their families and/or their communities is therefore now an important part of professional history. It allows historians to better understand personal motivations which in turn often reflect the social experiences of the age in which they are created.

WHERE CAN WE FIND HISTORY?

At a specialist level, history continues to be one of the most popular humanities degree programmes offered at universities in the UK. It provides skills in argumentation, presentation and problem-solving which make it a common route into law, teaching and management as well as into heritage-related jobs. The field of history remains a buoyant area for academic publishers. Professional historical societies, such as the Royal Historical Society and the Historical Association, can boast large memberships supporting their campaigns to promote the scholarly importance of the discipline. National, local, charitable and private archives, libraries and online repositories house the evidence of the past, be that in documentary, oral historical or material cultural forms. Very few of these repositories are closed to the public, which is part of the reason why even the most scholarly history can be regarded as an inherently democratic enterprise which can usually be accessed by those with an interest.

As for public history, we don't have to look far to find it. We only have to look around us to see that history saturates cultural and civic space and to understand why history is a mass activity as well as the profession of a few. Our cities and villages are full of architecture, statuary and commemoration which remind us of our past. Britain retains innumerable rituals and institutions which were started in periods long ago. But aside from living in a landscape that continually refers us to the past, we consume history hungrily, and in a variety of ways, as a leisure activity. History books regularly appear in the non-fiction bestseller lists; historical films and documentaries form the basis of a booming entertainment industry. Museums and heritage sites from the London Dungeons to (the rather more niche) Cuckooland Museum in Cheshire, England, draw in audiences from the UK and abroad. It appears that there is something for everyone. Popular cultural production involving history is immense, from the humour of *The Flintstones* (1960–1966) and *Blackadder* (1983–1989) to the glamorous intrigues of *The Crown* (2016–present) and *Bridgerton* (2020–present).

As will be discussed in Chapter 2, the history of health has a strong presence in this proliferation of representations – especially via popular and specialist books and articles, but also through TV shows, podcasts and blogs. As discussed in Chapter 4, many museums also deal principally with health historical issues, and a number of successful temporary exhibitions touching on health and wellbeing have confirmed the depth of the public appetite. We will discuss the implications and importance of these tangible areas where health and history are presented together for public consumption. However, the broader point to be made here is that history has moved a long way from being a specialised subject that was exclusively studied by elites. In the UK, the popularity of family history is a good case in point. Societies such as the Institute of Heraldic and Genealogical Studies and the Federation of Family History Societies act as important representative bodies nationally, but they represent only the tip of the iceberg in the popular area of family history which has abundant local forms. For example, the Anglo-Italian Family History Society, the Manchester and Lancashire Family History Society and the Caribbean Family History Group (covering the Midlands) are to name only three. In fact, as posited by Martin Bashforth (2012), family historians 'are probably the single biggest constituency of practising historical researchers within the wider public history community' (p. 203).[3] One needs only to go to The National Archives in Kew to see this popularity in action. It is demonstrated by pensioners digging out old war records and amateur historians sleuthing their family histories via national censuses and parish records. The excitement and enthusiasm in participation are evident in such historical immersion: touching the records and piecing together clues along archival pathways.

Of course, much family historical research these days can be pursued digitally from people's homes and there is less need for people to physically travel to archives. Vast genealogical databases can be accessed via websites such as www.ancestry.co.uk, www.findmypast.co.uk and www.myheritage.com. Significantly, these internet resources can help people trace ancestors, but increasingly also offer additional profiling services that can ascertain, from a quick DNA swab, our historic ethnic make-up and our predispositions to certain genetic disorders and diseases. Thus, these resources add a practical, diagnostic dimension to the 'usefulness' of history for health.

Lastly, history is not only consumed: it is constantly being created. Complex archiving processes go on in most large companies and institutions, and more historical evidence is created with every newly passed law, every minuted meeting, every parliamentary debate and the publication of every newspaper article or autobiography. The digital age has increased the possibilities of historical data capture exponentially, but also has created new problems, particularly in the vast quantity and range of data that is now produced. Should we keep every email sent? How long for? How will we ensure future technologies will be able to read artefacts from older ones? (Romein et al., 2020).[4] Digital archiving dilemmas to one side, at the level of the street, more and more people are actively documenting history as it happens, through photographs, blogs and vlogs. The majority of these forms of documentary evidence will be lost, but some will be retained, creating new resources for future researchers to interpret our present.

WHAT IS THE USE OF HISTORY?

The 'use' of history as a discipline that can (or should) be harnessed to improve the present is much debated. This discussion has been going on for over a hundred years but has yielded no definitive answers. It is nevertheless worth engaging with the debate here, not least because this book's remit – *history for health* – centrally implies some acceptance that the application of history is useful.

The usefulness of history has typically been expressed in expansive terms which emphasise history's provision of insights which extend empathy through the sharing of past experiences. In 44 BC, the Roman politician Cicero, in his essay reflections on old age, *De Senectute*, emphasised the satisfactions of later life and contemplated particularly on the way age gave people maturity and authority. He was saying, in essence, that by listening to old people, society would profit. This was because those who listened to the stories of older generations would be better equipped to avoid repeating similar mistakes themselves.

However, while examples of commentary touching on the perceived utility of history can be found as far back as ancient times, it has only been in much more recent times that the matter has become a centrally debated topic, discussed within scores of history books. On the one hand, many historians have argued strenuously against using the past to better understand the present, asserting that differences in contexts, and therefore meanings and values, make such comparisons virtually useless. On the other hand, other historians have powerfully argued that history nevertheless can provide an important template to help current and future generations navigate the benefits, limitations, challenges and opportunities of taking certain actions or approaches.

The camp that sees history as a targeted tool for understanding contemporary society and behaviour tends to be the smaller one, however, and is generally not in fashion. In 1968, historians such as Will and Ariel Durant argued for the importance of the past in illuminating present affairs. In their expansive overview of 5,000 years of world history, they argued that humankind has essentially been the same throughout history, despite superficial changes in the way different individuals and societies dress up and present their urges (Durant & Durant, 1968).[5] Allan Bullock (1994) similarly reasoned for the formative future-shaping potential of history, stating that 'the future is always open, never predetermined, and ... we can have a part in shaping it' (p. 19).[6]

While such prescriptive ideas rarely gain traction these days, modern historians are nevertheless increasingly comfortable navigating an important middle ground. They may stop short of a direct approach ('look at this in the past to stop this in the future') but they acknowledge that history can provide sources of comfort or alert us to possibilities we might not have otherwise considered.

The impetus for this openness to embrace learning history as a societally valuable pursuit comes from both within and outside the discipline. These days, particularly in the UK, arts and humanities researchers are under ever-swelling pressure to demonstrate the significance and reach of their research impact. This obligation has been brought into relief by the performance-based criteria of the Research Excellence Framework (REF) which has been in place as a measure of accountability for ongoing public investment in research since 2014. Meanwhile, there is increased governmental pressure on universities to show that non-vocational degrees are 'worthwhile' in terms of transferable skills and employability. These agendas have coalesced to put pressure on those teaching history within universities to justify themselves. In short, for better or worse, it is no longer perceived to be enough to present history learning as a self-indulgent antiquarian pursuit, or an intellectual exercise conducted for its own sake with no bearing on the present or the future.

Cautiously then, we are finding ways to articulate history's usefulness, while still being attuned to the inapplicability of modern judgements on past contexts. Historical empathy helps us to understand 'the common humanity we share with our forebears' (Tosh, 2015, p. 8) and gives us some consolation through recognition of situations and predicaments that are in some ways analogous to our own. Even when those situations differ in significant ways, they can still present us with frameworks for thinking through our own predicaments, by revealing responses or alternatives that we might not otherwise have encountered. It is my contention that we can benefit from these insights at the same time as understanding that the examples from the past would have been shaped by different social mores and world views.

One of the most striking books to show how things might have been otherwise is Theodore Zeldin's *An Intimate History of Humanity* (1995) in which Zeldin presents a history of the dynamics of feeling within human society. He presents a touching collection of case studies showing how people in different epochs and different geographical contexts have lost and regained hope, and navigated fear in their lives. He shows how conversation has provided comfort, how relationships between parents and children have been differently embodied, how individuals have overcome adversity and invented new ways to cope, and are continually redefining what it means to love. In essence, Zeldin is presenting his readers with an inventory of alternatives, using examples from histories to show the multitudinous pathways that might be taken. The stories inspire readers to go beyond the cultural and social expectations of the age in which they live and instead to reach into the historical past to imagine new ways of being. This view does not attempt to discipline readers in a prescriptive manner to learn from the 'lessons' of history, but subtly shows readers how they can draw inspiration from venturing beyond their familiar personal horizons, by showing how others have done so (Zeldin, 1995).[7]

HISTORY, HEALTH AND MEDICINE AS HYBRID DISCIPLINES

Having briefly described some important baselines about history, we should move to consider why history and health and medicine make such good bedfellows for an integrative study.

It is my contention that the two disciplines, far from symbolising two opposing cultures (the classical and the scientific, as famously described by CP Snow in his Rede Lecture of 1959), both break boundaries in remarkably similar ways. History is a 'hybrid discipline' straddling both arts and social sciences (Snow, 1959; Tosh, 2015, p. 43),[8] which to my mind makes it a perfect candidate for health improvement.

As touched upon above, history is narrative and subjective, but it is also evidence-based and objective. History seeks to uncover the 'truth' while recognising the existence of many truths, dependent on the evidence accessed. Furthermore, professional historians understand that any quest for discovery within the past is always coloured by the personal and societal preoccupations of the present, as expressed (often unwittingly) through the author. In the words of historian Ludmilla Jordanova (2019), '[t]here is no such thing as unbiased history, but there is such a thing as balanced, self-aware, history' (p. 5).[9] This acceptance of the central importance of objectivity amidst inevitably subjective creativity should be seen as history's strength rather than its hindrance. The duality, importantly for this book, positions history as an ally of healthcare and medicine because practice and application in that field of learning also sees disciplinary borders crossed.

Health and medicine, despite their modern-day reliance on data, evidence and proof, were conceived at their historical roots as the healing *arts*. Pre-modern (as well as much non-western) doctoring and caring engaged the patient and society holistically and saw no disconnect between drawing on a somewhat standardised armoury of therapies and embracing the idiosyncrasies of personal experiences of the treatments applied. Even today, in a world focussed on curative outcomes and featuring an abundance of remedial and palliative techniques, we find ourselves at a point where narrow reductionist readings of ill health are increasingly challenged. Clinicians and other caregivers regularly discuss the benefits of more integrated approaches to healthcare that move beyond narrow definitions of evidence-based medicine. For example, complementary or alternative medical (CAM) treatments such as acupuncture, chiropracty and aromatherapy have become popular. Holistic or CAM medicine has been a growth area for some time in the USA

(Horrigan, Lewis, Abrams, & Pechura, 2012) and, more recently, in the UK (see the National Centre for Integrative Medicine, Bristol).[10] A few CAM interventions, such as the Alexander technique, are even offered (albeit in a limited capacity) by the UK's National Health Service, and integrative medicine is seen by many as an important health pathway for the unwell.

Disease, furthermore, is understood these days as more than a biological entity. Taken to its logical conclusion, this idea signals the increasing acceptance that medicine relies on more than the natural sciences for its successful outcomes. Being unwell is a social and cultural experience integrating the natural, the social and the individual (Labisch, 1998, p. 7).[11] Although pathogens and germs might be organic entities with strict definitional criteria and to some degree predictable behaviours, the reactions that they induce in people are varied and particular, both physiologically and psychologically. Individual responses are shaped by each person's idiosyncratic tendencies and character, by people's political, social and economic contexts, and by how they situate themselves relative to performative expectations surrounding their gender, ethnicity, age and class. In short, it is *people* who thrust a discipline like medicine – built on evidence, rigorous analysis and statistical modelling – into unpredictable social worlds, populated with diverse responses and interpretations (Labisch, 2004, pp. 423–424).[12]

It is no linguistic coincidence that doctors, therapists and carers take detailed patient *histories* as part of their assessments for care. The structure and style of the case history have radically changed over time. As Nancy Tomes (1991) noted, case histories were increasingly becoming 'highly technical records crafted as much to avoid lawsuits as to document the course of individuals' illnesses' (p. 608).[13] Such trends have only grown stronger. Yet, the endurance of the case history points to its origins when the attending doctor needed to understand the patient's health from all perspectives, beyond just the sore arm, the unexpected lump or the unexplained fatigue which an individual might present. Patients telling their greater history – one of diet, habits, parentage, lifestyle and other health conditions, however subjectively or partially relayed – was (and to a large extent still is) the doctor's primary means of quickly capturing the patient's personal circumstances, present and past, as they assess how to proceed therapeutically.

Furthermore, modern medical advances – far from making things more straightforward – immerse society ever more deeply into complex ethical and social debates. Whether discussing IVF, abortion, gene therapy or euthanasia, the reach of the modern doctor, researcher or carer increasingly extends into the moral and ethical and the social. Medicine and healthcare therefore operate in a social context which endows them with broader social responsibilities, beyond the laboratory, clinic or bedside.

As the large role of psycho-social factors in determining health has become more widely accepted, social prescribing is enthusiastically embraced. As Chapter 4 will discuss, numerous projects have affirmed the importance of the arts and humanities in improving health outcomes and the experiences of being unwell or being a carer or being socially excluded (Saavedra, Español, Arias-Sánchez, & Calderón-Garcia, 2017).[14] However, while the agenda for social prescribing has engaged with the visual, performative and literary arts, history is less often explicitly referenced as an important tool. This is strange, because history is ubiquitous as an element of people's sense of self, family and community, but also because of the way history as a discipline is continually called upon at a national, even global, level. Furthermore, history has many commonalities with health and medicine. As disciplines, both are uncomfortable with being pigeon-holed because they embrace, at their core, the empirical and evidential *and* the creative and subjective.

THE SCOPE AND STRUCTURE OF THIS BOOK

Before we move on to the body of this book to look at examples of some of the most important ways history can be of help for health and wellbeing, I would like to address some of the book's limitations. First and foremost, the book only examines the westernised experience and often refers specifically to the UK context, largely because of the location of my life. I am limited by language to the Anglophone world, so while I have sought to include examples from other parts of the globe, I am mindful of the spatial confines of the book's contents. In offering a western-centric view, this work omits to include the connections between history and healthcare in non-western societies. This means the book does not explore how non-western societies have adopted western medical principles, or how they might use alternative means to engage their histories through traditional indigenous medical cultures, as expressed through storytelling or the passing of oral-historical information down the generations. While such a short work can never be definitive, it is still hoped that much of its contents will have wider applicability, or inspire thoughts, beyond my own particular precinct.

In a similar vein, history is a vastly popular subject. Even when homing in on the specific areas where health and history intersect, the field of examples for potential inclusion is massive. Books dealing with the history of health, illness memoirs and practitioner accounts, are too numerous to mention, as are campaigns by health activist groups and policy interventions. Museums, galleries, archives and case study exempla are also in impressive abundance. In all categories, I have drawn on just a very few examples, as it would be impossible to represent all the prominent and worthy work in these areas. My apologies to those I have been unable to include.

The book looks in turn at three main thematically organised areas where history has been shown to be useful for positive health outcomes: (a) reading, writing and doing history; (b) the role of history and historians in advancing policies and research and (c) history as a participatory community exercise, such as those located in museums and galleries, or via archaeological digs. I am sure readers and practitioners will find other ways that history supports health.

My task is to show historians, practitioners, carers and the interested public that there are many types of history and that an awareness of the meanings we attach to these different manifestations of history can be an important vehicle for health. Scholarly history, particularly the art of historiography, when rigorously undertaken gives people analytic tools to look critically at evidence and to question the objectivity of different sources of information. As such, it trains the mind in very much the same way as solving a puzzle or a crossword: piecing together clues to come up with an answer. But more than keeping us mentally agile, both public history and academic history help us to question our assumptions. In so doing, history extends our sympathies and enlarges our perspectives on how to deal with the modern-day problems (both commonplace and unique) that we face. History teaches us to appreciate moral courage, to visualise alternatives, and it can act as a timely reminder to those in difficult situations that their circumstances are unlikely to be permanent. Beyond helping us account for pain, history might also create new pains, perhaps in uncovering the hauntings of cross-generational trauma of our ancestors. Sometimes, engagement with history can also be used as a tool of resistance – particularly against the perceived power of the medical establishment and the authority of the medical gaze.

It has not always been easy in the past to make a case for integrating the arts and humanities with healthcare, but recent advances in the visual and literary arts have done much to raise people's consciousness and have produced many successful results. We have become broader in our approaches to being ill, which in turn have broadened and shaped our expectations about the kinds of care that we will find most useful and comforting. Additionally, for some time now, medical historians have signalled a slowly turning tide, highlighting the need to distinguish between the history *of* medicine and the role of history *in* medicine (Labisch, 2004; Sheard, 2008).[15] Twenty years ago, this was an aspirational entreaty. I believe that we are now at a point where the practical application of history to healthcare, while by no means yet routine, is no longer greeted with raised eyebrows as 'strange' or somewhat left-field. This shift, combined with the saturating power of broadcast and digital media, means that explicit recourse to history is around us today even more than it was in the past. Whether we are flicking through TV channels or browsing in a bookstore, history is a popular part of the daily bread and butter of our cultural consumption. We evoke it almost without thinking, as part of our reach for personal and collective meaning.

As history is deeply embedded in our personal, social and political worlds, it makes sense to interrogate the potential of the discipline's function for health and wellbeing. This book is a contribution to that inquiry.

NOTES

1. Butterfield, H. (1931). *The Whig interpretation of history*. London: G Bell & Sons.

2. Rosenzweig, R., & Thelen, D. (2012). The presence of the past: Popular uses of history in American life. In P. Ashton & H. Kean (Eds.), *Public history and heritage today: People and their pasts* (pp. 30–55). London: Palgrave Macmillan.

3. Bashforth, M. (2012). Absent fathers, present histories. In P. Ashton & H. Kean (Eds.), *Public history and heritage today: People and their pasts* (pp. 203–222). London: Palgrave Macmillan.

4. Romein, C. A., Kemman, M., Birkholz, J. M., Baker, J., De Gruijter, M., Meroño-Peñuela, A., ... Scagliola, S. (2020). State of the field: Digital history. *History*, 105(365), 291–312. https://doi.org/10.1111/1468-229X.12969.

5. Durant, W., & Durant, A. (1968). *The lessons of history*. New York, NY: Simon & Schuster.

6. Bullock, A. (1994). Has history ceased to be relevant? *The Historian*, 43(104), 16–19.

7. Theodore, Z. (1995). *An intimate history of humanity*. New York, NY: Harper Collins.

8. Snow, C. P. (1959). *The two cultures and the scientific revolution*. Cambridge: Cambridge University Press; Tosh, J. (2015, first published 1984). *The pursuit of history: Aims, methods, and new directions in the study of history*. Routledge.

9. Jordanova, L. (2019, first published 2000). *History in practice*. London: Bloomsbury Publishing.

10. Horrigan, B., Lewis, S., Abrams, D. I., & Pechura, C. (2012). Integrative medicine in America—How integrative medicine is being practiced in clinical centers across the United States. *Global Advances in Health and Medicine*, *1*(3), 18–94. https://doi.org/10.7453%2Fgah mj.2012.1.3.006. For the UK, see the National Centre for Integrative Medicine in Bristol https://ncim.org.uk or the Royal London Hospital for Integrated Medicine https://www.uclh.nhs.uk/our-services/our-hos pitals/royal-london-hospital-integrated-medicine.

11. Labisch, A. (1998). History of public health—History in public health: Looking back and looking forward. *Social History of Medicine*, *11*(1), 1–13. https://doi.org/10.1093/shm/11.1.1.

12. Labisch, A. (2004). Transcending the two cultures in biomedicine: The history of medicine and history in medicine. In F. Huisman & J. H. Warner (Eds.), *Locating medical history: The stories and their meanings* (pp. 410–431). Baltimore, MD: Johns Hopkins University Press.

13. Tomes, N. (1991). Oral history in the history of medicine. *The Journal of American History*, *78*(2), 607–617. https://doi.org/10.2307/2079538.

14. Saavedra, J., Español, A., Arias-Sánchez, S., & Calderón-Garcia, M. (2017). *Creative practices for improving health and social inclusion*. Seville: University of Seville Press.

15. Labisch, A. (2004). Transcending the two cultures in biomedicine: The history of medicine and history in medicine. In F. Huisman & J. H. Warner (Eds.), *Locating medical history: The stories and their meanings* (pp. 410–431). Baltimore, MD: Johns Hopkins University Press. See also: Sheard, S. (2008). History in health and health services: Exploring the possibilities. *Journal of Epidemiology & Community Health*, *62*(8), 740–774. https://doi.org/10.1136/jech.2007.063412.

2

READING, WRITING, RELATING, COLLECTING: THE HEALTH BENEFITS OF DOING HISTORY

As described in the first chapter, although history is in evidence all around us and we evoke it constantly, history (in its many myriad manifestations) is still not routinely regarded as a distinct part of the arts and humanities armoury to be mobilised for better health outcomes. This provides an interesting contrast to the practices of storytelling (Wilson, 2022) and reading (Davis & Magee, 2020) which have longer trajectories of praise for their benefits to wellbeing.[1] The side-lining of the discipline of history for health inspiration is itself symptomatic of history's cultural omnipresence. There is no doubt that we all take history so much for granted that most of us rarely pause to tease out and identify when we actively engage with it. The lack of recognition of the therapeutic potential offered by the practices of creating and relating history is particularly surprising because history is a literary art as well as a research method. History can be read, written or recited, lending it many of the same health benefits, one would think, as telling a story or reading or writing one.

Unlike the creative literary arts, however, history requires that the fount of historical narratives is rooted in interpretations of what *actually* happened. Rather than seeing this disciplinary require-ment as creatively restrictive, it can be argued that this solidity imbues history with additional discursive powers. In short, because history relies on reconstructing (even if in contestable ways) the reality of another individual, community or nation in different decades or epochs, each of its stories bears a powerful rubber stamp of authenticity. Having roots in actuality gives historical stories authority in ways beyond – or, to be more precise, different to – fictionalised accounts. In the realm of health, history narratives provide a portfolio of past experiences against which modern patients and practitioners can position themselves. It might be comforting to read about (or research) communities of people who have dealt with health conditions similar to one's own. It might be useful to understand how far therapies have come. It can offer insight to show how certain clusters of symptoms were classified, dealt with or experienced differently in the past. As people explore their health conditions, or as they investigate ways to look after those who are ill, historical accounts constitute the playbook of factual examples against which any current moment can be positioned.

This chapter will illustrate two major ways that carers, practitioners and patients can access history for health: first, through reading and writing it, at a scholarly or popular level; second, through the doing of historical research, whether this involves visiting an online or physical archive or taking oral histories (or being an interview subject themselves). This chapter refers to a large variety of academic and popular history books, details of which can be found in the suggestions for further reading in Chapter 6. That list contains just a few examples from within an enormous field of historical endeavour. It is meant to whet the appetite and encourage further exploration.

THE HEALTH BENEFITS OF READING AND WRITING HISTORY

Scholarly History

The history of health and medicine is a thriving academic subdiscipline. Many universities now offer modules on the history of health and medicine as part of their undergraduate history degree programmes, and master's level courses are numerous in the UK specifically and the global North more generally. Since the 2010s, health humanities have emerged as an important growth area, exploring not only the intellectual insights of cross-working between the health sciences and the humanities, but also specifically investigating how methods developed in the humanistic disciplines can be practically brought to bear on contemporary health experiences. Postgraduate-level health humanities offerings at University College London, University of York, University of Edinburgh, University of East Anglia and St George's, University of London – to name just a handful of UK-based examples – demonstrate a reassuring student appetite to explore this field. Many of these medical and health humanities degrees include components on literature, philosophy, political science, ethics and art as they relate to health and wellbeing, and all of the programmes, tacitly or otherwise, recognise the need for the students and future practitioners to understand development or stasis over time. This is also the case when the declared focus of a programme is to enfold real-world applicability into arts and humanities for health – for example, through the provision of modules looking at health communication, health policy and the application of the arts for health and social care more generally. There is no avoiding engagement with history.

Many of the scholarly history books written about health, illness, caring, trauma, marginalisation and dispossession fulfil an important social function. Some may have been written primarily as intellectual exercises, but many – I would argue *most* – also have an implicit (sometimes explicit) intention to advance and improve modern knowledge about health and wellbeing. This social mandate intrinsic to the writing of health history has always been evident to an extent but has been particularly clear since the blossoming of social and cultural history in the 1960s. It was at this point that increasingly large numbers of historians started to tell stories beyond the realm of the socially privileged: histories of women, children, minorities, workers and everydayness. Within the field of medical history specifically, the old-style grand narratives of medical inventions, discoveries and progress, typically written by elite, white doctors, began to give way to outputs produced by a younger generation of professional social historians eager to chart past social impacts and the experiences of health and welfare more broadly conceived. In the UK, groups such as the Society for the Social History of Medicine (est. 1970) led this change in focus. By the mid-1980s, the reorientation was in full swing when, in a now landmark article, Roy Porter called for medical historians to refocus their top-down gaze and instead think of writing history from the 'patient's view' (Porter, 1985).[2]

At the macro-end of the scale are histories of war, enslavement, genocide and systemic exclusion. While, on the face of it, these can be confrontational, harrowing histories, they do more than merely uncover and remind. They do restorative social work, helping to repair and build hope. In short, writing scholarly histories of tragedies or traumatic events can be beneficial for readers, particularly when they are members of the communities described. In this regard, one prominent area lies in Jewish writing about their historical experiences of repression and discrimination. Authors of many of these histories charting the evolution of antisemitism have actively framed their written contributions as embodying acts of consolation. To cite the stirring words of Rabbi Shim'on Bernfeld, a historian of Jewish experience whose *Book of Tears* presented the Jewish literary response to persecution from the era of the Maccabees to the nineteenth century: '[t]he stories of past woes are the future songs of consolation'[3] (Myers, 2018, p. 67). Other scholars have taken this theme further. David Myers' book *The Stakes of History* also deals with the writing of a history of Jewish peoples. According to Myers (2018), the consolations offered by history 'range from life-affirming to the lachrymose, from the self-effacing to the mocking, from the cyclical to the linear, and from the therapeutic to the obsessive' (p. 53).[4] Histories of slavery, colonialism, exploitation, violence and oppression can by extension be seen as achieving similar ends. Historical consolation offers new pathways for social cohesion and can provide opportunities for repair and rationalisation to communities after a major crisis or systemic trauma.

Although historians of Black or Jewish persecution, or indeed of any histories of minoritised groups are, sadly, still likely to have experienced discrimination in their lives, those who participate in writing their community histories today are unlikely to have had direct experience of many of the regimes, institutions and social contexts they describe. Yet, they live in the shadow of this history, a history which has left deep scars in the form of structural disadvantages or the endurance of repugnant social and cultural assumptions. In understanding how past people, institutions and policies created the structures, attitudes and cultures of the modern world, history can be the stimulus for new levels of collective and individual awareness-raising and introspection. With this social responsibility, history can work for keeping community consciousness alive and act as a vehicle for creating hope, developing courage and generating resilience for the future. For individuals and communities who have been misused or exploited by history, I would argue that engagement with history offers potential pathways for amelioration and movement towards more progressive attitudes.

Using this framework of history as consolation helps to bring the importance of academic medical and health histories into clearer focus. By interrogating former experiences and by pushing forward new interpretative understandings of diseases or lived conditions, historians can make relative assessments of attitudes today. These specialised understandings can then be passed on to the relevant communities in more easily digestible ways. As reflected by the author of a foreword to a recent book series on disability history essays: '[s]tudying disability history helps us resituate our policies, our beliefs and our experiences' (Anderson, in McGuire, 2020, p. ix).[5] The same argument could be applied to histories of any marginalised group: LGBTQ+ histories, women's histories, histories of people of colour.

Works dealing specifically with health history proliferate. The genre is too huge to mention all, but a few examples are listed in the final list of references and recommended reading within Chapter 6. Almost every major health condition or health event has its corresponding scholar historian. They include studies of specific diseases, such as cancer (Moscucci, 2016; Timmermann & Toon, 2012), tuberculosis (Bynum, 2015; Lougheed, 2017), HIV/AIDS (McKay, 2017; Weston & Elizabeth, 2022) and schizophrenia (Ophir, 2022). Others have looked beyond specific conditions to trace, for example, histories of pain (Bourke, 2014), histories of addiction (Courtwright, 2019) and psychiatric treatments (Scull, 2022). A large body of work is also focussed on the health histories of groups which were formerly socially ostracised: for example, histories of disability (Hutchison et al., 2020; Burch & Rembis, 2014; Durbach, 2010), transgender people (Heyam, 2022; Snorton, 2017; Stryker, 2017) and histories relating healthcare with race (Downs, 2021; Metzl, 2010; Reverby, 2009; Strings, 2019; Washington, 2006).

Furthermore, sophisticated retrospective critical analysis is not just the exclusive purview of historians. Critical theorist Susan Sontag's oft-cited 1978 book, *Illness as Metaphor*, on how metaphors for understanding and treating disease point to the victimhood of the sufferer, is just one example of a text emanating from outside the formal disciplinary boundaries of history but which centrally draws on numerous historical examples. In a similar vein, literary and linguistic studies of disease and illness narratives perform a special kind of history, where they unpick what was communicated and conveyed (and how). The far-reaching health benefits of these and other studies are not hard to grasp. For example, a 2009 exploration of how cancer is presented within novels, life-writing, drama and advertising, far from being a remote academic exercise, explicitly expressed the hope that its scholarly perspectives would bring context and meaning to those who were living with the disease (Schultz & Holmes, 2009, p. 3).[6] Academic studies, as well as being esoteric works demonstrating the intellectual gymnastics of members of the academy, can provide helpful underlying qualitative evidence that in turn can be translated for popular audiences to inform their health experiences, validating their importance and bringing insights to their current conditions.

For some of these authors, their interest in the subject matter was spurred by their own experiences of being unwell. Certainly, this was the case for Sontag. Although she never referred in her book to her own ongoing treatment for breast cancer, it was undoubtedly her reflections on her personal experience which caused her to write it. A study of women's health experiences by Elinor Cleghorn provides a more recent apposite example. In her preface to *Unwell Women* (2021), an ambitious work exploring the way women have been subjugated by the male medical gaze and diagnostic criteria, Cleghorn candidly admits that her historical research project was directly stimulated by her search for answers to her own illness (which turned out to be lupus). The writing of this history brought Cleghorn into an unexpected 'intimate kinship' with her subjects.

In Cleghorn's (2021) words, she felt that these women were 'part of my history. Their bodies contributed to the medical discoveries that meant my body recovered, and my disease could be managed' (p. 14).[7] Another powerful recent example, stimulated in this case by the author's experience of unexplained chronic seizures, is *Hysteria* by Katerina Bryant (2020).[8]

Popular Histories

While trained academic researchers can use their skills to critically excavate past histories of illness, disease, disability and trauma as they applied to certain groups – and so bring helpful health insights to readers and authors – it is imperative to note that health histories are not just of value when they are written by academic scholars. In recent decades, and particularly since the 1980s, people have started to research and write their own popular historical accounts of health. As well as being entertaining, largely because books of this type tend to be less heavy-going than their academic counterparts, these accounts have become popular resources to help people understand how the health context of the modern world came into being. But beyond that, these types of books are sought by individuals looking to connect their own intimate health experiences with those of others – a restorative practice of identifying a community.

The public appetite for health history is voracious. Popular page-turners cover an astonishingly wide array of health-related subject matter from major disease catastrophes in history, such as the fourteenth-century Black Death (Kelly, 2006), the 1854 cholera epidemic (Johnson, 2007), the 1918 Spanish flu (Barry, 2005; Spinney, 2017) and, most recently, COVID-19 (Chan & Ridley, 2021). Popular histories have also looked at single diseases over a long chronological period, offering a sweeping overview of the universality of human experience. One of the most sparkling examples is the Pulitzer Prize-winning *The Emperor of All Maladies*, an expansive historical account of cancer written by Siddhartha Mukherjee (2011), a physician and researcher in oncology. Other books take a biographical perspective. An expert in the popular biography genre is Lindsey Fitzharris, who has written two health-related bestsellers of this type: most recently, a biography of World War One plastic surgeon Harold Gillies (Fitzharris, 2022), and before that a work on the life and career of the pioneer of antiseptic surgery, Joseph Lister (Fitzharris, 2018). I would suggest that reading about the lives of doctors, nurses, carers and patients is such a popular area because being unwell is an archetype of the highly personal yet universal experiences that unite us all, irrespective of the cultures we are brought up in, or the time period.

However, within the realm of popular historical literature, it is the lived experience narratives that are the most heavily consumed by the public – and the subgenre is growing abundantly. These works bring micro-personal health histories to the table. The written style of these books is usually more immediately accessible and overtly empathetic than scholarly works, encouraging connectivity between author and reader, and helping to forge communities of health experiences across the customary restrictions of space and time. By way of a highly personal autobiographical voice, they reassure readers that they are not alone in their own struggles.

Again, I can select only the lightest smattering of examples from a field which is formidably large. At the end of Chapter 6 are references to books such as Tom Atkins' personal memoir of living with polio (1994), and powerful accounts of navigating life with a cancer diagnosis, such as those presented by Audre Lorde (1997) and Kate Pickert (2019). Additionally, I have included Christine Hyung-Oak Lee's (2017) account of her life after her devastating stroke and Porochista Khakpour's (2018) memoir of her journey to her diagnosis with late-stage Lyme disease, *Sick* (2018). The latter two are expressly mentioned because of the work they have done to widen the lived experience field to include narratives of illnesses that have traditionally received little coverage.

Unsurprisingly, mental health features strongly. Sathnam Sanghera's *The Boy with a Topknot* (2009) examines, often wittily and ruefully, some of the taboos of mental illness in his suburban family. More directly confrontational are eating disorder memoirs such as Marya Hornbacher's candid descriptions of bulimia and anorexia in *Wasted* (1998) and Portia de Rossi's frankly charted struggles with anorexia, as told in her 2010 book, *Unbearable Lightness*. Similarly popular are accounts of depression, bipolar disorder and anxiety. Three examples include *Underneath the Lemon Tree* by Mark Rice-Oxley (2012), *Haldol and Hyacinths: A Bipolar Life* by Melody Meozzi (2014) and *On the Edge: A Journey through Anxiety* by Andrea Petersen (2018).

Within this array of mental health memoirs, chronicles of addiction should be singled out for brief mention. These works have the oldest historical lineage and have laid the foundations for the current proliferation of authors revealing their private experiences to the wider reading public. The first success of this type can be traced back to Thomas de Quincey's *Confessions of an English Opium-Eater* (first published in *London Magazine* in 1821 and then a couple of years later in book form) describing both the pleasures and pains of laudanum addiction. The tradition continued through the twentieth century, demonstrated in Aleister Crowley's thinly fictionalised account of his heroin addiction, *Diary of a Drug Fiend*, published in 1922, and popular Beat Generation contributions such as *Junkie* (1953) by William Burroughs. Struggles with alcohol have been particularly prevalent in the genre. Examples include Jack London's *John Barleycorn: Alcoholic Memoirs* (1913), Chaney Allen's *I'm Black and I am Sober* (1978), former Arsenal captain Tony Adams' *Addicted* (1998) and the *Sunday Times* bestseller *The Unexpected Joy of Being Sober* (Gray, 2017). The list could go on.

But what does this mean? The increasing popularity of lived experience accounts describing journeys in health and wellbeing testify not only to the market hunger for the personal health histories of others, but also to the way these books are evidently useful to patients and care-givers today as they reach for the subjective experiences of others to help situate their own. These biographies, whether harrowing or triumphant in tone, provide windows into both more repressive and more permissive attitudes and behaviours. The collective exposure they provide confronts the silence and stigma which in the past has generally surrounded being unwell or traumatised.

Detractors might say that these are advice books dressed up as biographies (or perhaps vice versa) more than they are 'proper' histories, but I disagree. For sure, these lived experience authors do not envisage their works as history books in a formal sense, but they work as history in two major ways. First, they demonstrate the importance of writing personal histories for healing. These writers are united in viewing their literary production as catharsis, or at least a step along the road to emotional recovery or to acceptance. It is also apparent that these authors want their past stories to create meaning for others. The whole point of externalising their otherwise internal histories, therefore, is that they functionally provide social value beyond isolated experience. Here, we see writing for wellbeing in action, as both personal therapy and community care. Indeed, underscoring this view, life-writing has been described as scriptotheraphy.[9] Second, these lived experience accounts are history in that they provide important time-stamped testimonies. Every memoir therefore becomes a chronicle. These reminiscence narratives become a key constituent part of the published health archive of the future. They will speak as powerful subjective evidence to future historians of what it was like to live with X, Y or Z condition during the twentieth and twenty-first centuries.

As we move through the spectrum of historical literary making, from specialist academic works to popular paperbacks, it is worth mentioning as a short addendum the world of diaries. While some of these have been published, the most famous of all being the one kept by seventeenth-century Samuel Pepys (in which he frequently ruminated on his state of health between 1660 and 1669), others will remain in bottom drawers, far from public view. Most diaries will never be available as historical sources in the future, but their function is similar to writing a published lived experience narrative. Diaries are perhaps the most personal of all history books – and as such, deserve acknowledgement as important private sites of history for therapy or recovery and consolation. This is exemplified by the common practice of therapists asking their clients to keep a diary of their feelings, memories and personal histories.

This is not the place to talk in detail about all the other media pathways through which history reaches the public, but needless to say this examination of reading and writing history has elided the prominence of health histories in broadcast media and online. A whole chapter could be written on this alone. From television dramas and documentaries, films, radio shows and podcasts, to vlogs, blogs and TikToks, in our digital age people's health histories are around us more than ever. Revolutionary for its time, the BBC documentary *The Secret World of Sex* (1991) was one of the first to delve into 'private' stories using a format which presented ordinary people talking about their experiences. BBC radio shows such as *In the Psychiatrist's Chair* (1982–2001) and *The Listening Project* (2012–present) provide naturalistic, loosely structured forums which give listeners the tantalising impression that they are illicitly listening in to a private conversation. Podcasts from *Speaking for Ourselves* (2005–2006), a pioneering series spoken by people with cerebral palsy, to the immensely popular Radio 5 Live *You, Me and the Big C* (2018), featuring Dame Deborah James, demonstrate the public appetite to engage with oral testimony directly. As well as underscoring a shared desire to access private lives, these entertainments constitute crucial historical records of voices of the unwell, which can be consulted alongside, or instead of, evidence that has been written down.

THE HEALTH BENEFITS OF DOING HISTORY

To 'do' history is of course to write it, but in this section, I am particularly concerned with the research processes that lie behind the creation of any published or unpublished historical account. Both professional historians and amateur historians 'do' history. This might involve physically visiting an archive and laboriously sifting through boxes of documents; it might involve logging onto one of the many genealogy websites and starting to trace family origins via online census data or records of births, marriages and deaths. At a personal or familial level, doing history can be as simple as organising a family album, jotting down some notes about childhood, or putting together a memory box for future generations.

Most of this section will focus on oral history because this is the historical methodology which is regarded as holding the most direct therapeutic potential for its participants. It should be recognised, however, that the area where most people come into contact with the active application of the historical methodology is the area of family history. As mentioned in Chapter 1, family history brings research methods into people's quotidian lives, making active researchers out of casual consumers. Popular television shows such as the BBC's *Who Do You Think You Are?*, running since 2004, demonstrate the public's avid interest in genealogical stories. We will therefore start with family history.

Doing Family History

There is a vast array of guidance available on to how to conduct family history, but people usually start by searching for the sup-porting documentation that was produced at key points when citizens are forced to interact with the state: namely births, mar-riages and deaths. In the UK – similar to most places in the global North – this can be done relatively easily, using resources such as www.freebmd.org.uk (civil registrations in England and Wales) and www.gro.gov.uk (the website of the General Register Office) or, for Scottish descendants, the National Records of Scotland (www.scotlandspeople.gov.uk). Explicit health information in these records tends to be limited to an entry for cause of death on a death certificate, but it is these documents nevertheless which provide the stepping stones towards more detailed investigations. They help researchers find out people's former names, relation-ships, addresses and places of work – and, from this start, a pic-ture can gradually be pulled together of ancestors' lives. Sometimes these investigations throw up more complex journeys than might have been anticipated. Very much like a detective piecing together clues, once a hint of a particular life event is identified, the fam-ily historian can then follow it up and verify it, via more specific archival avenues. For example, some web archives allow search-es of former children's homes' resident lists (e.g. www.children-shomes.org.uk). Care and adoption records might be accessed via the Barnardo's 'Making Connections' application process (https://www.barnardos.org.uk/former-barnardos-children). The British Home Children Registry (http://britishhomechildrenregistry.com) can help to locate the records of British children sent to Canada as indentured farm workers and domestic servants between 1869 and 1939 (to 1948 for British Columbia). Convict transporta-tion records such as those listed at the Australian sister site to ancestry.com (www.ancestry.com.au) might help identify relatives who were deported to the Antipodes. Passengers' lists for ships,

housed at The National Archives in Kew, can be mined for emi-
gration stories. In the UK, donor conceived people born after 1991
are able to request information about their donor and genetic sib-
lings via the Donor Conceived Register run by Liverpool Women's
NHS Foundation Trust (https://www.liverpoolwomens.nhs.uk/our-
services/donor-conceived-register-dcr/).

Yet, while it is relatively easy to access the nuts-and-bolts
information, such as names and dates cited within government
bureaucracies, army records or ship passenger lists, the granular experiences of our ancestors' health are much harder to
piece together. The Hospital Records Database, accessed via The
National Archives, Kew (https://discovery.nationalarchives.gov.
uk), although not updated since 2012, provides many general
hospital records that can give contextual information, but individual patient files generally remain unavailable. Asylum records
contain other obstacles. Although admission and discharge regis-
ters do exist for most of these institutions, patients are typically
referred to by first name only. Furthermore, these hospitals did
not encourage either patients or staff to write diaries, memoirs,
poems or prose. Even in instances where these texts were produced, the institutions played no role in the retention of the materials. Consequently, almost no first-person accounts exist in these
archives. Nevertheless, some family historians do find the records
of former asylums useful. Large and well-known mental health
institutions such as Bethlem Hospital, Maudsley Hospital and
Warlingham Park Hospital can be accessed through the archives
of the Bethlem Museum of the Mind (https://museumofthemind.
org.uk/collections/archives), but there are several other less notorious institutions whose archives are usually placed within county
record offices.

In sum, for the interested and the persistent, there is a wealth of
archival opportunities for tracing family health stories, be they the
stories of orphans, the disposed, the sick or the bereaved. These in
turn can be supplemented with private material found in locked
attics or passed down through the generations. The emerging stories can be surprising in their revelatory capacities, but they just as
easily show themselves as quite ordinary. In either case, it is important for the historian researcher to remain critically open to the

possibility that they are only party to a certain version of any story. Even if a domestic history journey involves finding a box of letters indicating love between, say, a man and a woman, it should be recognised that '[t]he past was not all innocent and good', and families all undergo a process of 'content-ordering', editing out 'scandals and secrets' (Langellier & Peterson, 2004, p. 49).[10]

Because of the ways our family histories resonate with our personal identities, family researchers (professional or amateur) face a psychologically sensitive set of endeavours. A pertinent case in point can be seen in the published reflections on an intimate experiment conducted by Martin Bashforth when he used his training as a professional archivist to imagine being tasked to make up archive boxes for his grandfather, father and himself. Describing the process of choosing a selection of mementos and private memorabilia, Bashford (2012) quickly recognised that the choice was more than a pragmatic acquisitive process: it was also one that caused him to 'struggle with the emotions' (p. 206).[11] Similarly, I can vividly remember how confronting it was to clear out my parents' house when it became time to sell after they had both died. Returning to those familiar rooms, I found myself sorting through paperwork going back over decades. I also had the impossible task of weighing up the value of lots of seemingly inconsequential items. So many of the relics of their marriage had no particular meaning for me, but others offered glimpses of lives I had not really known. These fragments represented sides of my parents' younger characters to which I had never had access. The whole process took me on an intense emotional journey. This journey not only uncovered pieces of stories, but also made me question the validity of some of my own memories, and led me to realise how little I did know. Even though I am a professional historian, the process underscored how different histories could be constructed within the same family.

In some cases, the tracing of sadder and more disrupted histories, especially those that were long swept under the carpet and not talked about within families, can be therapeutic in providing long-sought-after answers. These are the common family secrets, the myth-making and the silences that can perplex younger generations or leave big question marks that cause anxiety and unease. However, it is necessary also to acknowledge that in other cases the discovery of settled happiness can provide a degree of comfort, perhaps precisely because of the ordinariness and everydayness uncovered. Actively doing family history gives all citizen researchers meaning beyond our own lives, providing a stronger 'sense of a much longer personal lifespan, which will even survive... death' (Thompson & Bornat, 1978, p. 2).[12]

Doing Oral History

It is an oral historical method, however, which has received the most praise for promoting positive therapeutic outcomes, although historians need to be careful not to over-promise therapeutic advancement given that they are not trained psychological specialists. Professional historians want to find out what happened, and therefore tend to view the health benefits of oral history as a by-product of their research processes, rather than their central goal. Amateur historians, however, may conduct oral histories for more explicitly emotionally restorative reasons. Once again, we find blurred boundaries. Both mental health practitioners and professional historians are invested in uncovering past narratives. Both facilitate journeys of personal acceptance through the contributions they offer, directly or indirectly, to psychotherapeutic healing.

The oral history method was born from a desire to uncover everyday histories, histories that are not necessarily recorded in an archive and might otherwise disappear without a trace. Since the late 1970s and early 1980s particularly, oral history has become increasingly nuanced and sophisticated in its analysis, working through themes such as the reliability and the subjectivity of memory, the power dynamic between interviewer and interviewee and the expectations unconsciously shaped by both the micro-level (room, building, atmosphere and city) and the macro-level contexts (time period, geographical location) of any interview. Perhaps the most influential work in recording experiences specifically within healthcare is that done by Joanna Bornat, Rob Perks, Paul Thompson, and Jan Walmsley (2000).[13]

Although the USA particularly has a strong oral historical tradition of recording 'great lives' – such as those of doctors, politicians and high-level bureaucrats[14] – oral histories of health have predominantly been collected from patients, carers and workers who customarily leave little trace in the archive.

Oral history democratises history: although oral evidence can be mediated and interpreted by professional historians, it can also be owned by the speakers and the communities themselves. Oral history interviewees often benefit from the value of being heard and are able to unearth memories which may have been buried for some time. The method is additionally useful in that it can provide a record of those who may not have the ability, or inclination, to write down their autobiographies. Recorded dialects and slang not only capture the grittier realities of past voices, but also serve powerfully to destigmatise difference and deconstruct myths of homogeneous identities. Having these voices incorporated can improve the self-confidence and sense of inclusion of the people recorded and may also serve a similar function for future listeners.

Although there are several ways to give an oral history, from long meandering storytelling responses to open-ended questions, to shorter direct answers to closed questions, it is generally agreed that naturalistic, non-prescriptive, free-form narrative produces the best results. Oral histories offer more than the articulated linguistic content – that is, they reveal a great deal more if the listener reflects on *how* the histories are told, as much as on *what* is said. As with all storytelling, the effective practitioner or historian should pay due attention to the pace, tone, gestures and silences that accompany any oral historical delivery. Moreover, oral histories, like stories, require mutuality. So, how a historical storyteller adapts their account (simplification, magnification and omission) for their listeners can also be highly revealing.

Therapy for the Oral History Subject
Specific contexts where oral historical recollection has been found to be beneficial are numerous and include application within trauma recovery, end-of-life care and within old age more generally. In these areas, the value is aligned to the benefits of talking therapy, although with oral history the focus must always include reflection on past events, without necessarily needing to relate them to

current ones. Of course, the historian who uncovers therapeutically useful information needs to be careful not to promise trained psychotherapeutic analysis. Nevertheless, it has been argued that in some situations 'the less "therapeutic" the goal, the more therapeutic the result will be' (Baum, 1981, p. 49).[15] Essentially, for a variety of complex reasons, people can be more happy to provide personal narratives in the service of the goals of history, than they are to invest in counselling or talking therapies.

There have been several studies which have looked to oral history as a method to help overcome trauma (Abrams, 2016; Cave & Sloan, 2014; Harvey, Mischler, Koenen, & Harney, 2000; Langer, 1993).[16] Sometimes this subgenre is referred to a crisis oral history. Survivor narratives range from the highly personal and individualistic to those involving collective responses to huge traumatic events of international importance. Perhaps one of the largest collections of narratives can be seen in Steven Spielberg's *Survivors of the Shoah* project, which gathered video interviews with nearly 55,000 Holocaust survivors between 1994 and 1999. Relatives of those interviewed in this project can request copies of their family testimony. On a more modest scale, but of no less importance, are smaller sample groups such as those accessed by Thomson (2015) to uncover the history of Fred Farrall, an Anzac survivor of the battle of Gallipoli in 1915.[17] An early example, slightly larger in scope, can be illustrated in the work of Hunt and Robbins in 1998 who described the value of narrative reconstruction in their study of World War Two veterans. Here it was shown that even though many of the interviewed ex-soldiers had hitherto been using tactics of avoidance of their war pasts, they nevertheless benefitted from articulating their histories. Furthermore, the framing of oral histories as information-gathering exercises, rather than as journeys specifically towards emotional retrieval, helped to capture stories from those veterans who otherwise might have been resistant to talking about the same experiences in an overtly clinical context. Nevertheless, for all those who took part, the participation reaffirmed the meaning and importance of their war involvement. It gave them agency to 'own' and shape their stories which *inter alia* became 'the most effective way of dealing with traumatic memory' (Hunt & Robbins, 1998, p. 62).[18]

Oral history for elderly communities is an area that enjoys widespread acceptance. One of the first studies was conducted in the 1970s when social anthropologist Barbara Myerhoff recorded in her book *Number our Days* the results of her living history classes for a community of elderly Jews in Venice, California. Myerhoff (1978) looked with humour at the roles that ritual and recollection could play in identity retention and reaffirmation, even as the body ages and the limbs and organs gradually fail.[19] At a broader social level, reflections on community histories such as these can shed light on populations that society often makes assumptions about, drawing out the authenticity and uniqueness of the lived experiences. Other studies have illustrated the therapeutic benefits of reminiscence for older people, be they through plays, poetry, writing or talking workshops or personal one-on-one conversations. These conversations, whether public or private, can affirm a person's sense of pride or accomplishment in their life; the reminiscence can confirm their kinship with others, or a sense of survivorship over more unpleasant events and experiences.

The elderly unwell are also identified as a group whose lives can be improved through oral historical engagement. In the UK, Joanna Bornat has done seminal work on oral history's usefulness for the elderly. Particularly innovative for the time was Bornat's development of a 'recall' reminiscence pack, in collaboration with the British charity *Help the Aged*, as part of *The Reminiscence Aids Project*, funded during 1978 and 1979 by the then Department of Health and Social Security. The concept was simple. Elderly patients with mental infirmities were gathered together and shown a sequence of images. The responses these triggered were then recorded. Although this became a popular activity in care homes, initial findings were inconclusive, partly because it was found that many of the organisers of reminiscence activities often excluded individuals who appeared to be the most unwell or disruptive. However, in terms of reaching out to aged groups, the impact on practice was profound and long-lasting. Since that time, Bornat's method has become an accepted practice utilised by psychologists, gerontologists and other care-givers for the elderly (Bornat, 1994, 2002).[20]

Some oral history studies have specifically targeted the improvement of the patient experience of dementia. Chaudry (1999), for example, homed in on reminiscence about places to help those with dementia regain a sense of selfhood.[21] Others have examined the method's utility in supporting dementia sufferers to access sporting identities (Russell, Kohe, Brooker, & Evans, 2019).[22] Even if the benefits are transitory and cannot change long-term health outcomes, oral history offers powerful moments of self-determination, working against social exclusion and giving a voice to those who otherwise would not be heard. The case study presented at the end of this chapter is a good example of one of these projects.

Beyond dementia care, work has looked at the role of oral history in end-of-life care, showing it to be a valuable tool for improving these experiences (Winslow, Hitchlock, & Noble, 2009).[23] Here, oral history is found to have an important agency-restoring function, helping even the very weak to be transformed from someone who has things done to them to someone who is in command of their own narrative.

Therapy for the Oral History Interviewer or Listener
Therapeutic gains are not just reserved for the interviewee. They can permeate to those conducting or consuming the oral histories, improving their practices or their mindfulness. By offering insights into what it is like to have a particular health condition, oral histories allow researchers, carers and clinicians to better understand illnesses and how they impact people in their everyday lives. This information can 'act as a springboard for the socialisation of entrants' into the health profession (Winslow & Smith, 2010, p. 386).[24] It can also expose injustices or inadequacies which can help to inform future strategies and directions.

Just as interview subjects are afforded kinship and comradery by their participation in oral histories, listeners to oral history testimony might relate the contents of an interview to their own lives and be comforted that certain experiences of health and illness are not unique. The benefits of this sense of kinship between speaker and listener are individualistic and non-uniform, but it does mean that people's relatable experiences can come into dialogue over relatively long chronological periods. For example, Helen Foster described her unpicking of the processes and feelings that she encountered when she used oral histories of former lace workers in the East Midlands as some of her inspiration for her historical novel. When approaching the recordings in a local studies archive, she had not anticipated that the process of accessing the histories would induce intense feelings of nostalgia which 'touches on the darkness in memories as well as uplifting moments in the past'). Foster explores the repercussions of what she calls 'eavesdropping' on the dead, as a positive source which inspired her fiction writing. For Foster, nostalgia created purposefulness. It became an inspiration for her creativity, as well as something that beneficially shaped the authenticity of her writing (Foster, 2020, pp. 104, 89).[25]

* * *

As I hope this chapter has shown, reading, writing and researching history can be a wonderful realm for psychological enrichment. This might be a deeply personal exploratory journey, the uncovering of a long-held family mystery, or the confirmatory solace of hearing and relating to the experiences of others. Whether the benefits derived are unanticipated consequences or the result of the historians' deliberate and directional intent, much of the work of historians – be they unwitting, amateur or scholarly – has a wellbeing and/or social improvement motive running through it.

Ten years ago, in a large American study, Rosenzweig and Thelen interviewed 1,500 people to illustrate the multiple ways people accessed history within their everyday lives. When the respondents reflected on the reasons why they engaged with history, they spoke in terms of its transformative potential to create a better society (Rosenzweig & Thelen, 2012, p. 51).[26] The study's findings are as relevant today as ever. Access to history belongs to all people, not just those educated to certain levels in the cultural hierarchy. The way we consume history, and the way we participate in history-making, permeates our lives. Doing history, whether by reading a book, telling a personal story from childhood, interpreting archival information or eliciting (or giving) oral testimony, helps us to feel better and helps us to care better by engaging with what makes us human. We question where we have come from to better equip us for where we are going.

CASE STUDY 1: ORAL HISTORY, HEALTH AND WELLBEING AND EVERYDAY LIFE WITH DEMENTIA

CHRIS RUSSELL AND GEOFFERY Z. KOHE

Description of Project

The lack of disease-modifying pharmacological interventions for dementia foreground the significance of research methods to support understanding of experiences of everyday life with the illness. Accordingly, this case study illustrates how oral history methodology might be mobilised for health and wellbeing and afford means to illuminate and advocate for individuals' voice within the health and social care sector. The case study draws data from a research project ('Because life's there ... understanding the experience and identity of people living with dementia in the context of leisure and fitness centres', 2016–2019) conducted in the UK involving four people (three men and one woman, all living with different forms of dementia causing illness, e.g., Alzheimer's disease, vascular dementia, etc.). The project aimed to understand experiences of regular engagement in physical activity, via their local leisure centre, with a specific emphasis on exploring ways involvement shaped participant identity. Cognisant of wider social and support networks, close family members and centre employees were included, if these individuals played roles in the experience of the person.

Methodology

Focussing upon the interpretation of human experience, the research took a phenomenological approach that enabled exploration of the physical environment, and ways bodily engagement informed expressions of meaning. Synergising with naturalistic and participatory methods (e.g. go-along interviews, where the researcher interacted with participants during physical activity), an oral history approach was used to foster participant voice and dialogue, and elucidate personal narratives of time and space. The methodology entailed participants connecting memories of the past to highly individualised (re)creations of their lives and experiences in the present. Emphasis was given in interviews and observations on using life histories to evoke memories that invoked conversation. A minimum of four interviews took place, with at least one encompassing the go-along method. The methodological value is highlighted in this example, taken from a go-along interview with Paul, a man in his late seventies living with Alzheimer's Disease, during a game of table-tennis. Paul laughed with the researcher as he headed the table-tennis ball and said, 'see, just like playing football!' Reminded of this at the end of the game Paul said, 'I was a centre half you know. My job was to save the team...you're on it most of the time'. This encounter expressed much about his identity and what physical activity meant for Paul's sense of self, then and now. The challenges Paul experienced with long-term memory and the worry this caused him meant he was inclined to say little. The go-along context, and historically focussed dialogue, however, enabled him to demonstrate techniques he used when playing football years ago, and afforded opportunity for reflection on that with clarity and insight.

To foster a positive and constructive dialogue, and enable individual's rich narratives to emerge, the oral history approach relied significantly on building rapport between researcher and participant. Beyond vital to the project's methodological rigour, rapport was paramount for ensuring ethical integrity and credibility of the research by ensuring participants' comfort with data collection. Additionally, the use of participants' own photographs – illustrating earlier sporting experiences – furthered rapport and encouraged detailed articulation of sporting histories. Recollections of close family members contributed accompanying context and insight. Ivan, for example, was a man in his early sixties living with a rare form of dementia, corticobasal degeneration, which impeded his verbal articulation rather than memory. When describing early experiences of sport (here playing football in the street as a child) he reflected, 'there's always people down there, whether it's you and your mates, or up or down from that you know ...'. His wife, Jemma, added, 'you played with your cousins as well didn't you? They used to say that he didn't mind being an only one because there was always someone round'.

Methodological challenges included the influence of nostalgia. However, an understanding of nostalgia offered ways of appreciating how links between the past and present influenced changing personal identity and emotions linked to sport participation. Excluding nostalgic recollection entirely therefore might have inadvertently denied individuals a core and legitimate part of their sporting story. Enabling a safe space for individuals to (re)create their own meanings and do so in ways that mattered to them was thus vital. Additional challenges were presented by the public nature of venues and participatory aspects of the research. For example, possible disclosure of personal information within a public venue (e.g. awareness others might gain that participants had dementia, if individuals wished this knowledge safeguarded), informing other attendees in the vicinity that research was occurring and ensuring consent to the researcher's presence. Here, rapport building enabled the researcher to understand whether a person felt comfortable about others knowing their diagnosis and assisted in developing appropriate explanation about the research. Rapport also facilitated curtailment of a go-along interview if the risk of inadvertent disclosure of personal information became acute.

Methodological Consequences and Lessons

An oral history approach offered means of exploring matters that were of personal importance to participants. Individuals were, specifically, able to reflect upon how involvement had changed over time and describe meanings and value they attached to their participation, identities and everyday lives. Findings and conclusions were made possible that may have been inaccessible using alternative methodological approaches. For example, as described above, where Paul elucidated upon earlier times in his life with feelings of happiness and confidence. In such ways, the project explored intersections between memory recollection, creation and first-hand experiences of participation in physical activity.

Utilising oral history, researchers could encourage participants to share aspects of their life story and consider how this mattered to their engagement and experience. Notwithstanding, there remains need to carefully consider the physical contexts/

settings in which the research takes place, as well as the nature and content of the discussion (and how these might evolve over time with rapport). Accordingly, we advocate for longitudinal-style oral history approaches that transcend 'snapshots' of individual's experiences, and allow evolution of thinking, recollection and meaning to develop, be challenged and remade over time. Thus, potentially, further crystallising richer accounts of experience than might initially be retrieved. Oral history helped bring to the fore the experiences of a group under-represented in sports history and wider health and social care historical literature. In taking the person's experience as central and accounting for contextual sensitives and sensibilities, the approach underscored the importance of an individual's biographical complexities and its inter- and intra-personal meanings. For example, here, how individuals have constructed their identities prior to, during and beyond the onset of dementia.

Suggested Pathways for Future Research

Adopting historical understandings of the sort described in this case study matters because numbers of people living with dementia continues to increase as populations age and people are being diagnosed at earlier stages in the disease trajectory. Recognition of what is offered verbally by participants must be complemented by an appreciation of communication made using other senses. In particular, the facial expressions of participants, their body language and tone of voice. An oral history approach beyond merely the oral may, thus, enable richer histories of identity, the body and participation.

New projects are already building from this initial research. An online educational initiative provided by the Association for Dementia Studies (University of Worcester, UK), Championing Physical Activity for People Affected by Dementia, involves practitioners from social care, health and housing, sports and leisure enhancing practice by working in concert to engage with accounts from people living with dementia participating in physical activity. Yet, more is required. For example, the issue of what constitutes good facilitation of physical activity for people living with dementia remains unresolved. Oral history can shed light on this link and amplify individuals' voices who may benefit the most from an enhanced provision, resourcing and participation.

NOTES

1. Wilson, M. (2022). *Arts for health: Storytelling*. Bingley: Emerald Publishing; Davis, P., & Magee, F. (2020). *Arts for health: Reading*. Bingley: Emerald Publishing.

2. Porter, R. (1985). The patient's view. *Theory and Society, 14*(2), 175–198. https://doi.org/10.1007/BF00157532.

3. Bernfeld, S. (1923–1926). *Sefer ha-dema'ot: me'ora'ot ha-gezerot veha-redifot veha-shemadot* (*The book of tears*, 3 vols.). Berlin: Hotsa'ot Eschkol, vol. 1, 147. Quoted in Myers, D. N. (2018). *The stakes of history: On the use and abuse of Jewish history for* life. New Haven, CT: Yale University Press.

4. Myers, D. N. (2018). *The stakes of history: On the use and abuse of Jewish history for life*. New Haven, CT: Yale University Press.

5. Anderson, J., in McGuire, C. (2020). *Measuring difference, numbering normal: Setting the standards for disability in the interwar period*. Manchester: Manchester University Press.

6. Schultz, J. E., & Holmes, M. S. (2009). Editors' preface: Cancer stories. *Literature and Medicine, 28*(2), xi–xv. Retrieved from https://www.muse.jhu.edu/article/402244.

7. Cleghorn, E. (2021). *Unwell women: A journey through medicine and myth in a man-made world*. London: Weidenfeld & Nicolson.

8. Bryant, K. (2020). *Hysteria: A memoir of illness, strength and women's stories throughout history*. Sydney: Newsouth Books.

9. One of the earlier texts to look at scriptotheraphy by that name was Henke, S. (2000). *Shattered subjects: Trauma and testimony in women's life-writing*. London: Palgrave Macmillan; Organisations such as Lapidus International act as communities of writers (some of whom

are historians) who support and promote the writing for wellbeing community (https://www.lapidus.org.uk).

10. Langellier, K., & Peterson, E. (2004). *Storytelling in daily life: Performing narrative*. Philadelphia: Temple University Press.

11. Bashforth, M. (2012). Absent fathers, present histories. In P. Ashton & H. Kean (Eds.), *Public history and heritage today: People and their pasts* (pp. 203–222). London: Palgrave Macmillan.

12. Thompson, P. with Bornat, J. (2017, first published 1978). *The voice of the past: Oral history*. Oxford: Oxford University Press.

13. Bornat, J., Perks, R., Thompson, P., & Walmsley, J. (Eds.). (2000). *Oral history, health and welfare*. Psychology Press.

14. Rivers (1967) is oft quoted as one of the first important oral histories of great men in the history of medicine. See Rivers, T. M. (1967). *Tom Rivers: Reflections on a life in medicine and science: An oral history memoir*. Cambridge, MA: The MIT Press.

15. Baum, W. (1981). Therapeutic value of oral history. *The International Journal of Aging and Human Development, 12*(1), 49–53. https://doi:10.2190/BYPE-EE50-J1TP-HV2V.

16. Abrams, L. (2016). *Oral history theory*. Oxford: Taylor and Francis; Cave, M., & Sloan, S. M. (Eds.). (2014). *Listening on the edge: Oral history in the aftermath of crisis*. Oxford: Oxford University Press; Harvey, M. R., Mischler, E. G., Koenen, K., & Harney, P. A. (2000). In the aftermath of sexual abuse: Making and remaking meaning in narratives of trauma and recovery. *Narrative Inquiry, 10*(2), 291–311. https://doi.org/10.1075/ni.10.2.02har; Langer, L. (1993). *Holocaust testimonies: The ruins of memory*. New Haven, CT: Yale University Press.

17. Thomson, A. (2015). Anzac memories revisited: Trauma, memory and oral history. *Oral History Review, 42*(1), 1–29. https://doi.org/10.1093/ohr/ohv010. This provides further reflections on his book: Thompson, A. (1994). *Anzac memories: Living with the legend*. Oxford: Oxford University Press.

18. Hunt, N., & Robbins, I. (1998). Telling stories of the war: Ageing veterans coping with their memories through narrative. *Oral History, 26*(2), 57–64. https://www.jstor.org/stable/40179522.

19. Myerhoff, B. G. (1994, first published 1978). *Number our days: Culture and community among elderly Jews in an American ghetto*. New York, NY: Plume.

20. Bornat, J. (Ed.). (1994). *Reminiscence reviewed: Evaluations, achievements, perspectives*. Maidenhead: Open University Press; Bornat, J. (2002). Oral history as a social movement: Reminiscence and older people. In R. Perks & A. Thompson (Eds.), *The oral history reader* (pp. 203–219). London: Routledge.

21. Chaudhury, H. (1999). Self and reminiscence of place: A conceptual study. *Journal of Aging and Identity*, 4(4), 231–253. https://doi.org/10.1023/A:1022835109862.

22. Russell, C., Kohe, G. Z., Brooker, D., & Evans, S. (2019). Sporting identity, memory, and people with dementia: Opportunities, challenges, and potential for oral history. *The International Journal of the History of Sport*, 36(13–14), 1157–1179. https://doi.org/10.1080/09523367.2019.1703690.

23. Winslow, M., Hitchlock, K., & Noble, B. (2009). Recording lives: The benefits of an oral history service. *European Journal of Palliative Care*, 16(3), 128–130. Retrieved from http://pascal-francis.inist.fr/vibad/index.php?action=getRecordDetail&idt=21730927.

24. Winslow, M., & Smith, G. (2010). Ethical challenges in the oral history of medicine. In D. Ritchie (Ed.), *The Oxford handbook of oral history* (pp. 372–392). Oxford: Oxford University Press.

25. Foster, H. (2020). At the Intersection of memory, history and story: An exploration of the nostalgic feelings that arose when listening to oral history archives as an inspiration for novel writing. *LIRIC Journal*, 1(1), 86–107.

26. Rosenzweig, R., & Thelen, D. (2012). The presence of the past: Popular uses of history in American life. In P. Ashton & H. Kean (Eds.), *Public history and heritage today: People and their pasts* (pp. 30–55). London: Palgrave Macmillan.

3

ADVISING, TESTIFYING, EDUCATING: HISTORY AS A CIVIC HEALTH RESOURCE

While the last chapter examined how history can improve health via public and professional participation, this chapter will take a slightly different perspective. It will examine how history can advance health and wellbeing when it operates through some of the main institutions or knowledge dissemination systems, of power within society. This approach may appear to prioritise a top-down perspective, but it is not so clear-cut as that. Agitation for change often comes from the grassroots of society: searches for health justice, better policy directions or improved health education can start via local, sometimes even personal, initiatives. I argue that history's potential to impact bigger societal issues is flexible and inspirational rather than prescriptive or limiting. History has a role to play as a civic resource which can be mobilised creatively to reshape some of the structures and attitudes within and around healthcare today. I explore this capacity by examining four powerful avenues through which history visibly works: within health policy, within health-related injustices, within medical and health education and as a symbolic rhetorical force for garnering support for a cause.

Some time ago the historian John Tosh (2008) explained in his book *Why History Matters?* that historical thinking helps to create 'critical citizens' (p. viii).[1] Tosh was one of the earlier historians to interrogate in depth the importance of history generally as a 'way in' to deliberate and inform modern-day public issues, but he was certainly not alone. As this chapter will show, since the 2000s, several other eminent historians, most notably Virginia Berridge, Sally Sheard, Julian Simpson and Stephanie Snow, have eloquently championed history's usefulness specifically for improving the delivery of healthcare policy. Others, such as Alix Green, have addressed the link between history and policy work more widely, beyond the realm of healthcare. This academic interest is both a response to and a symptom of increasing pressures to justify history as an impactful subject with real-world relevance. In this chapter, I draw heavily on this work, which has been foundational in setting up the subfield of history and health policy studies.

The policy-making arena, however, is not the only area where history has the potential for useful and far-reaching application. Historians have also been centrally involved in highlighting past inaccuracies or misrepresentations in the realm of health, so have had a tangible influence in bringing companies and individuals to justice through the provision of expert testimony. Furthermore, within the domain of education, historical teaching has also been advocated as useful within the content and delivery of tertiary health education and as a part of the continuing professional development provision offered to medical and healthcare professionals. Additionally, it cannot be ignored that history is regularly mobilised as a broader social force – a spur to stimulate political or attitudinal shifts in society. This latter point moves our focus again into the realm of public history. Symbolic recourse to history, while often emotive and rousing, relies less on the finely tuned granular insights of professional historians. Instead, history tends to be invoked in calculated, crowd-pleasing ways by those in positions of influence (politicians, lobbyists and group leaders) as a means of getting people behind a movement. This broad-brush approach might make the hairs on the backs of professional historians' necks stand on end – precisely because of the generalisations and romanticisation such evocations of history often embody – but in a chapter looking at history as a force for social change, it would be wrong to ignore this frequent deployment of the symbolic capital of history.

HOW CAN HISTORY BE USEFUL FOR POLICY?

By far the largest body of work arguing for what history can do to stimulate systemic change focusses on the role that professional historians can play in health policy-making. As mentioned in the first chapter, academic historians in the UK are now under more pressure than ever to show that their research has meaning and applicability within society. Reflecting the expanded performance measures to which arts and humanities staff in universities are subject, there is no doubt that much of the literature championing history's role in policy work is written by the historians themselves. However, it is worth noting that the traffic is not just one way. Within the policy-making field, examples do exist of individuals who have joined the chorus for the better integration of historical expertise into their workplaces.

The kind of history positioned as the most useful in the policy arena is that which can be provided by a highly trained professional historical expert. What this expert brings to policy circles is their critical analytical skills. These days professional historians are all generally agreed that history cannot predict the future, nor can it provide instrumental lessons for the present, but they nevertheless are eager to show the importance of their interpretative expertise as a means of critically analysing how current attitudes, or accepted axioms, came into being. In short, to use the words of Virginia Berridge (2016), historians offer 'policy analysis rather than policy prescription' (p. 120).[2]

Sometimes this process is called the 'past-proofing' of present policy work (Simpson et al., 2018)[3] – a notion that is the mirror of 'future-proofing'. Essentially, the process involves checking the robustness and rationale for historic actions, through looking at how precedents were handled, as a means of informing new directions. Past-proofing history is thus a method via which to challenge the central assumptions evident within policy frameworks. Furthermore, by revealing the strands of historical contingency, historians immediately serve to destabilise the present. In other words, by showing how things *might* have been different in the past, the historian simultaneously opens the possibility that things *might* be different in the present, and future, too.

Expert historians draw on different kinds of evidence which can be put to the service of policy development. They might offer archival research, whether for putting the record straight, nuancing current received views, accounting for certain perspectives or better understanding the structures and functions of organisations. They might also offer comparative analysis beyond temporal lines. For example, historians can show regional or demographic variations, or they might illustrate how experiences differ beyond national borders. Additionally, oral histories can provide insights into the roles of different actors and contexts in laying the groundwork for modern policies.

Although calls have become more frequent in recent years, the idea of using historians as specialist consultants for those working in policy-making circles is not entirely new. As Alix Green (2015) has shown, between 1965 and 1976, the UK's Treasury Department had a Historical Section whose remit was specifically to interrogate the past to shed light on modern proposals (pp. 28–29). Similarly, the Cabinet Office, Foreign Office, the Civil Service (via its policy lab) and MI5 all have long traditions of employing in-house historians to guide their policy work (Berridge, 2003, 2016, p. 118).[4] The value of historians' perspectives in this arena was recognised as early as 1968 in The Fulton Report, a government review of the Home Civil Service. The review identified that a fundamental weakness of the department was that it was staffed by generalists who were spread too thin to meaningfully possess the expertise needed in all areas to look holistically at any given issue. The Fulton Report recommended a programme of modernisation, framed as professionalisation and rationalisation, which rested intrinsically on calls to give civil servants access to a wider pool of experts in the conceptualisation of their policy work (Green, 2015, pp. 28–29).[5]

Although the 'use' of historian experts has been acknowledged, if patchily, for some time, there has not been a sustained or proactive drive to include historical perspectives in policy-making. The exception to this is the History and Policy network (https://www.historyandpolicy.org) founded in 2002. In the UK at least, this has become the most important initiative linking historians with policymakers. It provides a forum for historians to present their research in the form of opinion pieces. Once reviewed, these expert pieces are disseminated by the History and Policy press officers, who purpose-fully stream them towards the relevant policymakers, government departments and journalists. As Sally Sheard (2018) has described, this is a 'bespoke' bridging service, the fruits of which have been pub-lished on the 10 Downing Street website or have been referenced in parliamentary inquiries.[6] As even a cursory scan of the History and Policy website shows, the range of themes on which historians feel able to comment is extensive: from business and finance, to farming and food, to trade unions and employment. Notably, papers relating to medicine and health are always prominent.

HOW HAS HEALTH HISTORY BEEN USEFUL FOR HEALTH POLICY?

Within the specific realm of health policy, the integrated use of historians has been slowly growing. Although the Department of Health still has no regularly employed historians, it has expressly drawn on historical consultants for their input into public health initiatives. An early example of this occurred in the 1980s when the Chief Medical Officer, Sir Donald Acheson, chaired an inquiry into public health reforms to which historians gave evidence. Also, during the 1980s and 1990s, as a prominent historical researcher in the history of drugs and public health, Virginia Berridge (2003) became a regular advisor to policymakers on drugs, alcohol and AIDS policies.[7]

Sally Sheard's public health work provides one of several instructive examples. Sheard worked with the local government in Liverpool in 1997 to generate discussions on the changing determi-nants of public health in the region. One of the major public-facing outputs of Sheard's project was a large exhibition at the Museum of Liverpool Life. This exhibition was not only conceived as public entertainment but it was also used as political leverage to raise awareness among local councillors and National Health Service (NHS) authorities concerning the impact of reduced public health spending (Hamlin & Sheard, 1998).[8] The success of this undertak-ing acted as a springboard for Sheard to become involved with a larger project in the early 2000s which saw her working closely with the then Chief Medical Officer, Liam Donaldson, to critique how expert medical knowledge had often been side-lined in favour of fiscal or politically expedient priorities. The ensuing publication, *The Nation's Doctor: The Role of the Chief Medical Officer, 1855–1998* (Sheard & Donaldson, 2006), has subsequently been used and cited by parliamentarians and journalists as one of their spurs to argue for key staff to be better trained in the use of expert advice in public health matters.[9]

The list of examples could go on. Historian Pamela Cox (2013) has described her experiences working as a youth justice consultant in Vietnam and a lay member of a local Family Justice Council in East Anglia.[10] Julian Simpson and Stephanie Snow have more recently circulated their results from a collaboration with GPs and health policy professionals to better understand the historical determinants shaping the current character of policy investigations into patient access to GP care (Simpson et al., 2018).[11]

However, even when their advice is not explicitly solicited, and they are not working in a formal collaboration, historians can be a vocal bunch. There are numerous illustrations of powerful commentary by historians on health-related matters where their articulate advocacy, even if not actively sought, has reached government ears. Many of these examples have been highlighted in Berridge's work. One was a powerful 1986 editorial by the medical historian Professor Roy Porter in the *British Medical Journal* calling for the liberal, non-punitive treatment of AIDS patients. The article, provocatively entitled 'History says no to the policeman's response to AIDS', generated sufficient interest in governmental circles that members of the Ministry of Health were quickly on the phone to the Wellcome Unit where Porter then worked, keen to hear his views as to how government responses should be moderated. In a similar vein, an article in *The Guardian* in 2001 on the foot-and-mouth cattle epidemic, written by (now Professor) Abigail Woods while she was still a history Ph.D. student, was important for stimulating widespread debate over the action which the government should take during that well-publicised public health crisis (Berridge, 2003, p. 514).[12]

Since the inception and subsequent flowering of the History and Policy network, the trend of historians offering health policy advice has intensified and become more purposefully targeted on specific issues. The examples are too numerous to mention more than a few (full details are in the reference list at the end of Chapter 6), but prominent opinion pieces include Matin Gorsky's (2006) presentation of evidence of pre-NHS community involvement in hospital governance; Ali Haggett's (2016) call to bring male mental health higher up the agenda of a governmental task force report on mental health; Siobhán Hearne's (2021) efforts to destigmatise sexual health disorders; and Coreen McGuire's (2020) searing exposure of digital exclusion within the welfare system for disabled and poor citizens.

Most recently, papers stimulated by the public health emergency ushered in by the COVID-19 pandemic have, unsurprisingly, been popular. Historians have offered insights concerning, for example, how to respond to misinformation and conspiracy theories about COVID-19. Using History and Policy as their dissemination platform, Fox, Coast and Forward (2022) made recommendations, based on their historic findings, that the government would be wise to change the tone of their public health campaigns. On the same topic of pandemic response, a group of medical historians have posited that insights gleaned from citizens' behaviour during the Blitz could usefully inform COVID-19 public health strategies (Irving et al., 2020). While historical advice typically relates to fairly recent periods of modern history, on occasion even historians with a pre-twentieth-century focus have found ways to proffer valuable advice. A good example is Hugh Small, an expert on Florence Nightingale. Small argued in 2020 that the best way to maximise local resources in public health campaigns against COVID-19 may be to devolve to local authorities the powers of decision-making and financing of epidemic control, as was customary in the nineteenth century in Nightingale's era (Small, 2020).

Oftentimes, however, historical research is not written with an explicit policy-changing intention in mind but has proved important in exposing sticky or problematic histories. These histories in turn come to bear on public consciousness, creating a snowballing effect whereby they rise up the government's agendas and come to impact future policy directions. Perhaps the most striking example of this is in the published historical research surrounding the tobacco industry's reaction to the link between smoking and lung cancer, as established by medical researchers from the 1950s. History books such as Allan Brandt's *The Cigarette Century* and Robert Procter's *Golden Holocaust* powerfully exposed the story that the American cigarette industry knew full well the health risks of their products, and yet still actively strategised how to market them (Brandt, 2008; Proctor, 2011). This side of the Atlantic, historians such as Berridge (2007) have also interrogated the tobacco story, uncovering the 'corporate relationship' that the British tobacco industry evidently enjoyed with the government.[13] Building on these important foundations, the field of tobacco history continues to grow with recent work examining the role that sports sponsorship has played as a vehicle to circumvent advertising restrictions on tobacco. As my own work has shown, even though cigarette advertising was banned on UK television in 1965, the cigarette industry actively explored other ways to advertise its products and even went so far as to lobby (behind the scenes) the then Minister for Health not to impose additional restrictions (O'Neill & Greenwood, 2022).[14]

As we shall shortly discuss, these prominent exposé histories had such an impact that they sometimes even brought historians into the courtroom. Other works, however, have also been important in influencing policy change because of the gravity of the evidence they uncovered. Pioneers in this area include two historians of occupational health, Arthur McIvor and Ronnie Johnston, who in 2001 published their interviews of 31 people who had worked with asbestos between 1940 and 1990. These oral histories created a vivid picture of the way asbestos exposure had impacted the health of individuals and families. Evidence from this historical survey was then mobilised as part of the national campaign to ban asbestos in Scotland which lobbied government to bear some responsibility for the high asbestos death toll 'because of the sheer inadequacy of workplace regulation' (Johnston & McIvor, 2001).[15]

Happily, the clarion call for more history experts in the policy forum does not just come from the side of the historians themselves. In recent years, members of the health sector have also joined the chorus championing the benefits of taking on board a serious historical analytic approach. Public health specialists have drawn attention to the need for history in professional identity formation, as well as professional development and communication, and have passionately advocated for history's central importance to the effective conduct of public health research.

Some public health researchers have been directly critical of the ahistorical tendencies of their discipline. They have argued persuasively that ahistoricism is particularly troublesome for public health professionals, given that public health represents the branch of scientific endeavour that is most deeply embedded in broader political, social and environmental contexts. Furthermore, they argue that public health is a subject that can benefit from longitudinal studies spanning several generations, as it needs to be able to understand the contextual drivers for progress, or lack of progress, when public health plans have been tested and applied in the past.

Access to the sometimes-divergent motivations behind different national responses to seemingly similar health challenges also provides an analytical frame. Although such frames might be more readily grasped by investigators trained to understand historical contingency, they can also be immensely helpful to public health workers. A good example of how history has been mobilised to support comparative policy research can be found in an American study looking to understand why the majority of the country's public health professionals have taken a particular stance on e-cigarettes. To understand the dynamics, the public health authors of the study have called for the need for a better understanding of the historical trajectories which underpin the current position in different nations. In England, Public Health England (PHE) and several anti-tobacco charities have taken a harm reduction perspective when framing their advice on e-cigarettes. While these bodies agree that e-cigarettes are not perfect, and indeed can still produce harm, this harm is regarded as less than that produced by cigarette smoking. This pragmatic response contrasts with the position generally followed in the USA. Here the national stance holds no room for exploring the role of e-cigarettes in reducing tobacco harm. Instead, public health bodies in the USA have almost all taken a much harder line, favouring outright abstinence. The study concludes that it is only by taking a comparative historical perspective that each nation's modern standpoint can be understood as being in line with their past political responses to addictive substances, from the early twentieth century onwards. Only once this is recognised does the English harm-reductionist position, contrasting with the USA prohibitionist attitude, make sense (Green, Bayer, & Fairchild, 2016).[16] This sort of innovative research, stimulated from within the public health sector itself, sets the stage not only for predicting future national positions on other similar issues but also points to ways to modify those positions. It is this critical historical perspective which affords contemporary commentators a first step towards exploring future options.

The key to effective integrative history and policy-working of course relies on good communication and a willingness by people working in different fields, often with dissimilar immediate objectives, to be open to ways of thinking that might not be typical within their daily working lives. Part of the onus here lies with professional historians, to make their art accessible and easily digestible. Historians need to simplify their language, broaden their appeal and start to think a bit more practically about how to translate their research. Equally, stakeholders in politics, policy and the media need to better grasp the central point that historians are not offering the lessons of the past. The value of historian experts in healthcare is their critical historical approach with its unique set of interpretative tools which can be applied to past knowledge and actions. These can in turn provide more nuanced and insightful understandings of the past, a subtly different (but arguably richer) offering than any promise to provide direct and instrumental answers for the present.

HISTORIANS IN THE COURTROOM

As an extension of policy work, we now turn to the role that historians can play in the courtroom, particularly as expert witnesses, but also in terms of raising awareness of issues which stimulate legal redress. Taking a bird's eye view, the historian's role within legal scenarios is quite unsurprising. Like lawyers, one of the central tasks of the professional historian is to probe and review evidence and judge if there are alternate narratives which might be claimed and can be supported by the evidence. Even if the historian was not present at the original events, their discipline trains them to bear witness to the past. Historians, in short, are authoritative experts who can be brought in precisely to test and reinterpret the accounts of others.

In the American context, where there has long been a more developed litigious culture than in Europe or Australasia, there is a tradition of utilising historians for their expert opinions within explicitly legal settings. The longevity of this phenomenon is surprising, with examples as far back as the 1950s of historians supplying courtroom evidence, notably within a landmark civil rights case *Brown* v. *Board of Education* (1954) (Rothman, 2003).[17] Turning specifically to health-related matters, perhaps one of the largest legal trials that called on historical evidence was the revisiting of the US Public Health Service (USPHS) Tuskegee syphilis experiments (1932–1972). The subject of these now infamous trials was the USPHS-commissioned study which examined how untreated syphilis advanced in its African American participants. These participants were not fully informed of the treatments they were given or why (being told they were being treated for 'bad blood'). Furthermore, even though from 1943 syphilis was largely curable with penicillin, many Tuskegee participants were denied treatment because the purpose of the study prioritised charting the full progression of the disease. This major ethical and racist scandal led to a number of court cases, the most significant being a class-action lawsuit filed on behalf of the study participants and their families, which resulted in a $10 million out-of-court settlement in 1974. Several experts presented evidence in this trial, including those involved in medicine and public health, but also historians who were able to uncover through archived material the way the study was conducted and how participants had been systematically misinformed (or uninformed). The case attracted much media attention and was not only successfully defended in favour of the study's subjects, but President Bill Clinton acknowledged the wrongdoings in a public apology in 1997.

This example was by no means exceptional, however, and there are several other cases of health litigation cases being won through the presentation of compelling historical evidence. Work by Gerald Markowitz and David Rosner exposed the 'deceit and denial' of the American chemical and lead industries, drawing on meticulous historical research to prove how to paint manufacturing businesses failed to act on information in their possession about the cancers and other health problems associated with working in their industries. Their work moved beyond an exposé within the pages of an academic history book. In fact, the historians who found the incriminating evidence in the archives proceeded to become closely involved in the provision of legal testimony against the paint industry, bringing justice for unsuspecting lead-poisoning victims (Markowitz & Rosner, 2002; Rosner & Markowitz, 2019; Whitehouse, 2019).[18]

Analogously, professional historians were employed by both plaintiffs and defendants in the 1990s and 2000s when several cases were raised alleging that the tobacco industry knowingly misled the public about the health risks of tobacco smoking. Some of those historians, such as Robert Proctor and Allan Brandt, testified against the tobacco industry in different American court cases, arguing that the industry had denied, hidden or manipulated information regarding smoking's carcinogenic effects in order to protect sales. However, over 30 historians, most prominently Kenneth Ludmerer, former president of the American Association for the History of Medicine, provided expert witness testimony in defence of the tobacco industry (Maggi, 2000; Proctor, 2004).[19] This involvement has raised a series of ethical issues. Proctor and Brandt have questioned how appropriate it is to have health historians testifying in a manner that does *not* act in defence of public health.[20] Proctor (2012), ever vocal, has gone so far as to say that the historians who offered evidence in support of the tobacco industry should themselves be called to account for being implicated in spreading 'the world's deadliest malignancy' (p. 91).[21]

Although the calling of historians to courtroom settings is most prevalent in the USA, this is not to say that the phenomenon is absent from other national contexts. For example, in a series of tribunals organised in 1975, historians of New Zealand were asked to be expert witnesses to determine the ownership of land claimed by the Māori population under the 1840 Treaty of Waitangi (Belgrave, 2012).[22] In the UK, there was a prominent trial exposing human rights violations and physical and mental cruelty inflicted by British soldiers on Kenyan Kikuyu populations during the Mau uprisings from 1952 to 1963. In 2009, Leigh Day commenced a legal action in the High Court in London representing several victims of the uprisings. This trial brought historians such as David Anderson and Caroline Elkins into court to show how evidence had been systematically covered up and left hidden for years after the events. Once again, historical evidence helped to decide the verdict and, in 2013, the British Government was forced to offer £19.9 million in compensation to over 5,000 claimants who had suffered abuse during Mau.

In a similar vein, historians have helped in enquiries to bring psychological peace to those who suffered abuse at the hands of individuals wielding celebrity status and power. The most high-profile of these cases was the 2015 trial of British TV presenter, Jimmy Savile, who systematically sexually abused dozens, potentially even hundreds, of people in 28 NHS hospitals over several decades while working as a TV star and charitable philanthropist. In the legal enquiries mobilised against him, which were only pursued after Savile's death, it is notable that historians were asked to provide some of the contextual evidence. This historical data and perspective helped to shape an independent report into the failings of the NHS which was prepared for the Secretary of State for Health in 2015 (Lampard & Marsden, 2015).[23] The report fed into the landmark criminal investigation into Savile by Scotland Yard, resulting in Savile being posthumously stripped of many of his honours and the NHS being compelled to pay damages to 52 of Savile's victims.

It is not just the professional historians who gather the most compelling evidence, however. Sometimes historical evidence emerges 'from below', particularly in the form of oral testimony from the victims themselves. This evidence becomes especially impactful when it is curated in such a way that it is given wide exposure through public release and dissemination. One of the earliest ground-breaking moments where the oral history was demonstrated to stimulate change and legal action was in 1998 with the release of the documentary *Sex in a Cold Climate* by Testimony Films. This film charted the sexual abuse that unmarried mothers were subjected to within Catholic Magdalen 'laundries' (homes) in

Ireland. When it was broadcast, the film provoked an outpouring of corroborative testimonies. As such, it presents a powerful example of how oral histories have been used to publicly expose crimes of the past. In the case of *Sex in a Cold Climate*, the film opened the floodgates for other stories documenting abuse in Irish Catholic homes, stimulating numerous legal actions and raising public awareness further through the release of a 2002 Miramax film, *The Magdalene Sisters,* directed by Peter Mullan.

HISTORY WITHIN HEALTH EDUCATION

Simultaneous with these developments is a strong current of work which argues for the importance of history to be included within the standard training offered for health, medical, public health and other caring professionals. This takes us back to the view expressed in Chapter 1 that health and history are not as far apart as might be indicated by snap judgements presuming the oppositional categories of 'sciences' and 'arts and humanities'. Certainly, there is interest among health professionals to read historical perspectives, not least because many medical and healthcare journals have history sections as part of their regular offering. In the global North, *The Lancet,* for example, has a routine 'Art of Medicine' essay, and the *American Journal of Public Health* and *The American Journal of Health Promotion* also have regular history features. Special issues of the *British Medical Journal* have similarly centred on historical themes.

Promoting engagement with history, however, goes beyond just making historical perspectives available for interested or incidental reading by those working in professions aligned with health and wellbeing. It is increasingly argued that history should be integral to how health professionals are trained. The rationale draws on the benefits which can be derived through 'historical empathy', which was a movement within education which began in the second half of the twentieth century in history and social science. Using techniques of historical empathy, *feeling* as well as thinking is encouraged in historians (or wannabe trainee historians). This approach humanises historical research, not only by helping historians to better understand why past actors acted as they did but also through actively reminding historical researchers that they are humanly affected by their subjective feelings on any matter. Historical empathy can be taught in a variety of ways including detailed work with primary sources, first-person essay assignments, the use of documentary film and the integration of reflection into any form of instruction.

Historical empathy as a tool of education centrally involves 'student identification of diverse perspectives, analysis of the historical context of documents, and the making of affective connections to content' (Perrotta & Bohan, 2020, p. 599).[24] Highly relevant to our focus on health and wellbeing, Baron and Levstik (2004) supplemented previous definitions of historical empathy by adding a conceptualisation of empathy as *care*. In short, they argue that history students should not be detached, non-judgemental observers, but should be actively encouraged to care about people and events of the past. In this way, they can recreate imaginatively what it *must have been like* but also have a means of accessing past notions of caring in order to change future attitudes and behaviours (Baron & Levstik, 2004).[25] The core idea here is that historical empathy not only makes better historians who can identify with the contemporaneous constraints and world views available to historical subjects at the time, but it also makes them into specialist ambassadors that understand care and nurture in different time periods.

Beyond its application in the teaching of history, historical empathy is also being discussed more in the realm of health and medical education. Here, powerful arguments have been put forward that even subject areas as temporally remote as classical literature can contribute fruitfully to the development of empathy in medical students and practitioners (Kampourelli, 2022).[26] Furthermore, medical students themselves have perceived the advantages of drawing on real cases stored within their own history banks of emotive and formative experiences. This sort of recourse to history can capture (and guide) a different set of professional responses than what might otherwise be mobilised through the standard teaching provision of lectures, examinations or demonstrations. Simply expressed: the use of real experiences drawn from history offers the important reminder that compassionate care and medical treatment are sometimes different things.

Although the surge of approval for historical empathy in health-care teaching settings is quite recent, the insertion of history into health and medical curricula is not a new movement. As early as 1926, German surgeon Ernst Ferdinand Sauerbruch (1875–1951) strongly advocated for university medical students to be taught history. For Sauerbruch, it was imperative that his students understood

> *that medical science is culturally bound and hovers up and down alongside the trends of time (…) Therefore: History of medicine [is] not as an end in itself, but in connection with the living act of healing. (Labisch, 2004, p. 419)*[27]

One of the core reasons why health history is relevant is that health is determined by contextual factors above and beyond the immediate disease environment or the personal (genetic, chemical) susceptibilities of an individual. Health is shaped by much broader structural social, economic and environmental determinants. As Baruch has argued, history should be seen as a 'low-technology tool'. It is only

> *[b]y taking students out of their comfort zones and encouraging them to think critically and creatively about medical practice, [that] maybe we will provide a generative space for them to understand their place in it. (Baruch, 2017, p. 43)*[28]

Other studies have found that teaching medical students a credit-bearing medical humanities module as part of their clinical education has directly resulted in improved empathy, which in and of itself has been related to improved medical outcomes (Graham et al., 2016).[29] This can be regarded as a significant benefit, not least because other studies have shown empathy to decline in practicing physicians, often due to factors such as burnout (Hojat, Erdmann, & Gonnella, 2013).[30]

Perhaps slightly more surprisingly, sites of material collections of history – medical museums – have been identified as valuable locations in which to advance medical education, even if some of the specimens and collections might seem somewhat old-fashioned, even morbid, to modern students. These material collections allow students to channel learning through their senses via up-close interaction with tissues, organs and samples. While this interactivity might produce a visceral reaction, it also has the benefit of connecting the goals of the student with the goals of doctors of the past. This perspective does not deny the usefulness of newer, more digitally ambitious forms of teaching (such as virtual reality and multimedia-based methods), but it re-inserts the value of historical artefacts in teaching as a means of extending the empathy of medical students. Medical museums become more than just another way to observe the progress of disease or to illustrate unusual phenomena; they become sites for capturing nature's diversity and for posing questions about the effects of social and epistemological contexts (Marreez, Willems, & Wells, 2010; Wakefield, 2007, p. 380).[31]

As argued by Scally and Womack (2004), history also should be positioned at the heart of professional public health training:

> History consigned to the margins may be able to do nothing, but public health practitioners equipped with insight and understanding about the impact of political and social developments on the evolution of public health practice are better armed to fight the many skirmishes that still lay ahead in the battle to improve population health. (p. 753)[32]

Although there has been no wholescale change making history an essential element of all public health training, certain public health degrees have sprung up in the UK which have applied components that invite historical contributions. Some master's degree programmes in public health, such as those offered by the London School of Hygiene and Tropical Medicine or the University of Liverpool, are two prominent examples of 'science'-orientated degrees embodying an integrative approach with history.

HISTORY AS A SPUR TO CHANGE OR A CALL TO ACTION

A chapter examining the role of health history to improve health and wellbeing within civil society would be incomplete without a brief mention of the strategic (albeit sometimes haphazard) application of public history in high-profile media or political declarations. Here my interrogation is less about whether the historical comparisons drawn are historically watertight, or would ever be made by a professional historian, but instead focusses on the potency of history to stimulate change or call people to action, in ways that advance health-improving behaviours. Of course, history is all around us, and instances of companies, charities and individuals calling on history to promote their causes are too numerous to mention. Indeed, once you start consciously looking, it is clear just how common the references to historical precedent are. From Malcom X, to Gandhi, to Mandela, history has been routinely evoked as a spur to change.

Looking specifically at the promotion of health, the most obvious recent example can be seen in the way historical precedents were called upon in COVID-19 reportage. Particularly, it was commonplace for media representatives and policymakers to make comparisons with the flu epidemic of 1918 or the avian swine flu pandemics of more recent times. Journalistic articles in prominent media outlets, ranging from *The Guardian* newspaper in the UK to *Time* magazine in the USA, have made repeated non-specialist, but nevertheless highly compelling, comparisons between behaviours and responses to earlier epidemics and those of the coronavirus pandemic. In terms of savvy political rhetoric, it was no accident that the UK's Conservative government named the emergency hospitals opened in response to COVID-19, as 'Nightingale' hospitals. This purposeful reference to Florence Nightingale operated as a clever image management exercise, as it closely aligned a national heroine of past health history to a modern public health response. Prime Minister Boris Johnson's public relations team even encouraged him to record a short rousing video, talking about nursing history, on International Nurses Day in May 2020, as a means to stimulate national pride during a time of domestic and international crisis. History in this context became the way to galvanise political support and raise spirits at the peak of the pandemic. Rather than focussing on the restrictions on freedom of movement that the virus had necessitated, speeches like this one instead focussed audience attention much more positively on a tribute to the modern-day members of the nursing profession who provided the majority of front-line health support.[33]

Johnson's speech is of course just one example, but it rests on a long tradition of alluding to the past to underscore policy positions or to highlight, through historical comparison, the contemporary achievements of a government or shadow government. A brief search through parliamentary speeches reveals just how often the past is evoked within Westminster. In the last 75 years, one of the most cited historical moments in the realm of health was the founding of the NHS in 1948. There have been countless parliamentary mentions of lobbyists and politicians (both left and right-wing) ardently harking back to Nye Bevan's original vision of the NHS, as a means of powerfully situating their arguments about the health challenges within the present world.

Harnessing the symbolic force of history to mobilise new attitudes or push through new policies is not just the territory of journalists and politicians, however. Certain public health advocacy organisations such as Action on Smoking (ASH) actively use history in framing their campaigns. Downloadable information packs, such as *Key dates in tobacco regulation, 1962–2020* (available on the ASH website) illustrate how health charities and campaigning groups regularly draw on historical events and narratives as a means of bringing modern-day challenges into focus.

* * *

There is, of course, a profound difference between the fine-grained analysis done by professional historians and the general elicitation of history as used for drumming up public enthusiasm in newspapers, in parliament and on soap boxes. This is not in dispute. But whether we turn to expert historians as vital 'enlightened sceptics in the knowledge economy' (Cox, 2013, p. 126),[34] or resort to history as part of a rousing speech or call to action, the social function of history and its capacity to be mobilised to improve health situations cannot be denied.

History cannot provide direct answers or prescriptive advice, but it can help those in positions of influence to raise their gaze. History can embolden those who have their eye on civic health improvements, as it offers them a powerful vehicle to help policymakers, educators and politicians to navigate the political, social and organisational structures of our time.

Within this analysis, and perhaps not surprisingly given my day job, I argue that it is the work the professional historian can do in a society which is particularly exciting. Historical experts can be utilised in numerous ways. They can uncover new evidence, and in so doing, they can restore voices to dialogues which had previously excluded them. History can critique the way prophets and propagandists have manipulated attitudes in the past to get supporters for their causes. History can provide options that might be usefully deployed in new health and wellbeing contexts, but it can also provide reassurance, through the weight of experience, that new healthcare directions might not be as frightening or revolutionary as those implementing them might fear. In short, historians can offer those shaping the health of modern society – whether as health policymakers, justice seekers or educators – both the familiarities and contradistinctions of the past. They provide an interpretational and analytic tool kit to spot gaps, rectify silences, debunk myths and open the inventory of alternatives for those whose jobs involve the challenging task of purposefully navigating a healthful present.

CASE STUDY 2: DISABILITY HISTORY FOR
EQUITABLE FUTURES

COREEN MCGUIRE

Description of Project

Disability historians have a particular responsibility to apply their historical research to the present and investigate its relevance to ongoing lived experiences. While disability history's use for personal wellbeing and health may vary with the individual researcher, it should be central to policy development and can provide crucial impetus and evidence to make broader structural changes. Disability historians must look backwards and forwards. In what follows, I discuss how I put this mandate into practice by developing the health policy implications of a 2019 article on the use of spirometry in historical investigations of miners' lungs. Spirometers assess vital capacity by measuring exhalatory ability – thus enabling the proxy measure of 'vital capacity' or lung capacity. The development of this measure was key to the Medical Research Council's (henceforth MRC) interwar investigation of miners' lungs in South Wales. Although their efforts successfully legitimated the existence of a miner's lung as a disease resulting from coal dust, the threshold the MRC used to establish normal lung function was taken from a baseline measurement of working miners. This meant that compensation was denied to miners with lived experiences of breathlessness because the standard for normal lung function was artificially lowered in this group due to racist and classist biases.

Methodology

My examination of the MRC's 1942–1945 investigation of pneumoconiosis in South Wales miners involved extensive analysis of published scientific reports alongside testimonies from miners and doctors held in the National Archives, UK, the South Wales Miners Library and the University of Bristol's Special Collections. My historical research was shaped by my collaboration with the wider *Life of Breath* project; a multidisciplinary Wellcome funded project that explored new ways to think about breathlessness and demonstrated that arts and humanities approaches could ease the distress connected to long-term breathlessness.[35] One of the key preoccupations of the project was the challenge of measuring breathlessness and the frequent disjunct between objective and subjective measures of breathlessness.

Findings

By investigating the historical development of these measures in the context of mining, my article demonstrated that seemingly objective measures of health developed in conflict with subjective testimonies of lived experience. The MRC successfully established that disease due to coal dust was negatively impacting coal miners' respiratory health – as the miners had long asserted. However, the MRC's attempts to correlate the lived experience of breathlessness to quantifiable levels of respiratory disablement through spirometry rested on a flawed standard. The spirometer's production of useful numbers was critical for the development of diagnosis classification and corresponding compensation levels. Yet, the spirometric standard used in the investigations to represent normal lung function was determined using data from apparently healthy miners rather than a non-mining control group, meaning the standard was what was 'normal for miners' (McGuire, 2019a).[36]

Lundy Braun was the first person to use rigorous historical research to establish that the use of race correction factors in spirometry was biased. Her work showed that the use of race corrections has legitimated the assumption that differences in lung capacity between the races are due to biological factors, thus obscuring and diminishing the relevance of living standards and the impact of racism on health. This kind of thinking is dangerous because it ascribes differences between groups to the essential constitutions of its members rather than ways of living as a member of that group (McGuire, Macnaughton, & Carel, 2020).[37] As a result, we focus on the individual rather than considering the impact of their environment. We cannot change individual biology or personal risk factors but there is much that policy changes can do to modify the environment and decrease social and economic inequalities.

Indeed, the idea that white lung function is normal lung function has continued to negatively impact compensation for non-white claimants today (Braun, 2014).[38] Nevertheless, I was surprised when my close reading of the MRC investigation raised the possibility of a 'Welsh racial factor' to support the investigators' categorisation choices for data classification. This idea in part justified the idea that miners were a separate category with separate data requirements and standards of health. This assumption meant that miners' lived experiences of breathlessness were denied when they attempted to obtain compensation for a respiratory disability. Their testimony was considered inferior to measurement technologies that were elevated as objective. My article concluded that technology interacts with welfare provision to elevate 'mechanical authority over subjective experience for explicitly political ends' (McGuire, 2019a).[39]

Possible Health Policy Implications

I developed the finding that technologies can enable and amplify political biases in a 2020 *History and Policy* report which reasoned that our faith in the 'relationship between symptom experience and measurement' is flawed and that scientific objectivity has been wielded to 'systematically deny benefits to the disabled whilst maintaining the pretence of fairness in assessment' (McGuire, 2020).[40] These findings were further incorporated into the *Life of Breath* project's policy report, which recommended that 'Healthcare training and education should integrate a biomedical understanding of breathlessness with an experiential view, seeing it as an experience akin to pain'.[41] In *The Lancet Respiratory*, I further argued that this history illuminates the urgency of amplifying the voices of those with lived experience in current medical practices (McGuire, 2019b).[42]

The calls to stop using race as a variable in clinical algorithms have increased during the COVID-19 pandemic and have explicitly cited 'the long, rotten history of racism in medicine' to justify its exclusion (Vyas, Eisenstein, & Jones, 2020).[43] One 2022 article in *Chest* considered pulmonary function testing and argued against the practice of using race or ethnicity in medicine to explain differences between individuals and proposed changes in interpretation strategies to reduce health disparities (Bhakta et al., 2020).[44] It cited my article.

In conclusion, disability history that engages with the lived experience of historically marginalised groups can have broad-ranging health benefits that go far beyond the individual researcher. Disability history methodologies must be combined with politically motivated activism and its relevance must be recognised and sought out by policymakers. In this way, disability history can shape equitable futures.

NOTES

1. Tosh, J. (2008). *Why history matters*. London: Palgrave Macmillan.

2. Berridge, V. (2016). History and the future: Looking back to look forward? *International Journal of Drug Policy, 37*, 117–121. https://doi.org/10.1016/j.drugpo.2016.09.002.

3. Simpson, J. M., Checkland, K., Snow, S. J., Voorhees, J., Rothwell, K., & Esmail, A. (2018). Adding the past to the policy mix: An historical approach to the issue of access to general practice in England. *Contemporary British History, 32*(2), 276–299. https://doi.org/10.1080/1 3619462.2017.1401474.

4. Berridge, V. (2003). Public or policy understanding of history. *Social History of Medicine, 16*(3), 511–523. https://doi.org/10.1093/ shm/16.3.511; Berridge, V. (2016). History and the future: Looking back to look forward? *International Journal of Drug Policy, 37*, 117–121. https://doi.org/10.1016/j.drugpo.2016.09.002.

5. Green, A. (2015). History as expertise and the influence of political culture on advice for policy since Fulton. *Contemporary British History, 29*(1), 27–50. https://doi.org/10.1080/13619462.2014.953485.

6. Sheard, S. (2018). History matters: The critical contribution of historical analysis to contemporary health policy and health care. *Health Care Analysis, 26*(2), 140–154. https://doi.org/10.1007/ s10728-017-0348-4.

7. Berridge, V. (2003). Public or policy understanding of history. *Social History of Medicine*, *16*(3), 511–523, 516. https://doi.org/10.1093/shm/16.3.511.

8. Hamlin, C., & Sheard, S. (1998). Revolutions in public health: 1948, and 1998. *British Medical Journal*, *317*, 587–591. https://doi.org/10.1136%2Fbmj.317.7158.587.

9. Sheard, S., & Donaldson, L. (2018, first published 2006). *The nation's doctor: The role of the Chief Medical Officer 1855–1998*. CRC Press. For a discussion of the use of this historical research, see Sheard, S. (2018). History matters: The critical contribution of historical analysis to contemporary health policy and health care. *Health Care Analysis*, *26*(2), 140–154. https://doi.org/10.1007/s10728-017-0348-4.

10. Cox, P. (2013). The future uses of history. *History Workshop Journal*, *75*(1), 125–145. https://doi.org/10.1093/hwj/dbs007.

11. See Note 3. https://doi.org/10.1080/13619462.2017.1401474.

12. Woods, A. (2001, February 28). Kill or cure? *The Guardian*. Discussed in Berridge, V. (2003). Public or policy understanding of history. *Social History of Medicine*, *16*(3), 511–523. https://doi.org/10.1093/shm/16.3.511.

13. Berridge, V. (2007). *Marketing health: Smoking and the discourse of public health in Britain, 1945–2000*. Oxford: Oxford University Press.

14. O'Neill, D., & Greenwood, A. (2022). "Bringing you the Best": John Player & Sons, cricket and the politics of tobacco sport sponsorship in Britain, 1969–1986. *European Journal for the History of Medicine and Health*, 1-33. https://doi.org/10.1163/26667711-bja10022. Accessed on August 11, 2022.

15. Johnston, R., & McIvor, A. (2001, June 8). *Oral histories of the asbestos tragedy in Scotland*. International Ban Asbestos Secretariat. Retrieved from http://ibasecretariat.org/eas_rj_am_scotland.php.

16. Green, S. H., Bayer, R., & Fairchild, A. L. (2016). Evidence, policy, and e-cigarettes—Will England reframe the debate? *New England Journal of Medicine*, *374*(14), 1301–1303. https://doi.org/10.1056/nejmc1606395.

17. Rothman, D. J. (2003). Serving Clio and client: The historian as expert witness. *Bulletin of the History of Medicine*, 77(1), 25–44. https:// doi.org/10.1353/bhm.2003.0035.

18. Markowitz, G., & Rosner, D. (2013, first published 2002). *Deceit and denial: The deadly politics of industrial pollution* (Vol. 6). Oakland, CA: University of California Press; Rosner, D., & Markowitz, G. (2019). An enormous victory for public health in California: Industries are responsible for cleaning up the environments they polluted. *American Journal of Public Health, 109*(2), 211–212. https://doi.org/10.2105/ ajph.2018.304887; Whitehouse S. (2019). A lead-abatement judgment driven by science, history, and the law. *American Journal of Public Health, 109*(4), 544. https://doi.org/10.2105/ajph.2019.304983.

19. Proctor, R. (2004). Should medical historians be working for the tobacco industry? *The Lancet, 363*, 1174–1175. https://doi.org/10.1016/ s0140-6736(04)15981-3; Maggi, L. (2000). Bearing witness for tobacco. *Journal of Public Health Policy, 21*(3), 296–302. Thirty was an estimate made by Proctor in 2004, so the number is likely to be significantly more than that now.

20. Proctor, R. (2004). Should medical historians be working for the tobacco industry? *The Lancet, 363*, 1174–1175. https://doi.org/10.1016/ s0140-6736(04)15981-3; Brandt, A. M. (2004). From analysis to advocacy: Crossing boundaries as a historian of health policy. In F. Huisman & J. H. Warner (Eds.), *Locating medical history* (pp. 460–484). Baltimore, MD: Johns Hopkins University Press.

21. Proctor, R. N. (2012). The history of the discovery of the cigarette–lung cancer link: Evidentiary traditions, corporate denial, global toll. *Tobacco Control, 21*(2), 87–91. https://doi.org/10.1136/ tobaccocontrol-2011-050338.

22. Belgrave, B. (2012). Something borrowed, something new: History and the Waitangi Tribunal. In P. Ashton & H. Kean (Eds.), *Public history and heritage today: People and their pasts* (pp. 311–322). London: Palgrave Macmillan.

23. Lampard, K., & Marsden, E. (2015). *Themes and lessons learnt from NHS investigations into matters relating to Jimmy Savile*. Independent report for the Secretary of State for Health. Retrieved from

https://assets.publishing.service.gov.uk/government/uploads/system/uploads/attachment_data/file/407209/KL_lessons_learned_report_FINAL.pdf.

24. Perrotta, K., & Bohan, C. H. (2020). Can't stop this feeling: Tracing the origins of historical empathy during the Cold War era, 1950–1980. *Educational Studies*, 56(6), 599–618. https://doi.org/10.1080/00131946.2020.1837832.

25. Baron, K. C., & Levstik, L. S. (2004). *Teaching history for the common good*. London: Routledge.

26. Kampourelli, V. (2022). Historical empathy and medicine: Pathography and empathy in Sophocles' Philoctetes. *Medicine, Health Care and Philosophy*, 25, 561–575. https://doi.org/10.1007/s11019-022-10087-y.

27. Quotation from Ferdinand Sauerbruch translated and quoted in: Labisch, A. (2004). Transcending the two cultures in biomedicine: The history of medicine and history in medicine. In F. Huisman & J. H. Warner (Eds.). *Locating medical history: The stories and their meanings* (pp. 410–431). Baltimore, MD: Johns Hopkins University Press.

28. Baruch, J. M. (2017). Doctors as makers. *Academic Medicine*, 92(1), 40–44. https://doi.org/10.1097/acm.0000000000001312.

29. Graham, J., Benson, L. M., Swanson, J., Potyk, D., Daratha, K., & Roberts, K. (2016). Medical humanities coursework is associated with greater measured empathy in medical students. *The American Journal of Medicine*, 129(12), 1334–1337. https://doi.org/10.1016/j.amjmed.2016.08.005.

30. Hojat, M., Erdmann, J. B., & Gonnella, J. S. (2013). Personality assessments and outcomes in medical education and the practice of medicine: AMEE Guide No. 79. *Medical Teacher*, 35, e1267–e1301. https://doi.org/10.3109/0142159x.2013.785654.

31. Wakefield, D. (2007). The future of medical museums: Threatened but not extinct. *Medical Journal of Australia*, 187(7). https://doi.org/10.5694/j.1326-5377.2007.tb01304.x; Marreez, Y. M. A. H., Willems, L. N., & Wells, M. R. (2010). The role of medical museums in contemporary medical education. *Anatomical Sciences Education*, 3(5), 249–253. https://doi.org/10.1002/ase.168.

32. Scally, G., & Womack, J. (2004). The importance of the past in public health. *Journal of Epidemiology and Community Health, 58*(9), 751–755. https://doi.org/10.1136/jech.2003.014340.

33. Ward, E. J. (2020, May 12). Boris Johnson pays tribute to 'today's Nightingales'. *LBC News*. Retrieved from https://www.lbc.co.uk/news/uk/boris-johnson-pays-tribute-to-todays-nightingales/. Accessed on May 12, 2020.

34. Cox, P. (2013). The future uses of history. *History Workshop Journal, 75*(1), 125–145. https://doi.org/10.1093/hwj/dbs007.

35. Project findings are available at www.lifeofbreath.org. The team was led by Principal Investigators Havi Carel (University of Bristol) and Jane Macnaughton (Durham University).

36. McGuire, C. (2019a). 'X-rays don't tell lies': The Medical Research Council and the measurement of respiratory disability, 1936–1945. *British Journal for the History of Science, 52*(3), 447–465. https://doi.org/10.1017/S0007087419000232.

37. McGuire, C., Macnaughton, J., & Carel, H. (2020). The color of breath. *Literature and Medicine, 38*(2), 233–238. http://doi.org/10.1353/lm.2020.0015.

38. Braun, L. (2014). *Breathing race into the machine: The surprising career of the spirometer from plantation to genetics*. Minneapolis, MN: University of Minnesota Press.

39. McGuire, C. (2019a). 'X-rays don't tell lies': The Medical Research Council and the measurement of respiratory disability, 1936–1945. *British Journal for the History of Science, 52*(3), 447–465, 462, 465. https://doi.org/10.1017/S0007087419000232.

40. McGuire, C. (2020). How technology has been used to deny benefits to the disabled. *History and Policy*. Retrieved from https://www.historyandpolicy.org/policy-papers/papers/how-technology-has-been-used-to-deny-benefits-to-the-disabled.

41. More than a medical symptom: The need for holistic care of breathlessness (2018). *Policy Report, 43*. Retrieved from https://www.bristol.ac.uk/policybristol/policy-briefings/life-of-breath/.

42. McGuire, C. (2019b). Dust to dust. *The Lancet Respiratory Medicine,* 7(5), 383–384. https://doi.org/10.1016/S2213-2600(19)30116-X.

43. Vyas, D. A., Eisenstein, L. G., & Jones, D. S. (2020). Hidden in plain sight—Reconsidering the use of race correction in clinical algorithm. *The New England Journal of Medicine, 383,* 874–882. https://doi.org/10.1056/NEJMms2004740.

44. Bhakta, N. R., Kaminsky, D. A., Bime, C., Thakur, N., Hall, G., McCormack, M., & Stanojevic, S. (2022). Addressing race in pulmonary function testing by aligning intent and evidence with practice and perception. *Chest, 161*(1), 288–297. https://doi.org/10.1016/j.chest.2021.08.053.

4

TOUCHING, VISITING, DIGGING: PARTICIPATORY HISTORY FOR HEALTH

Moving away from history's role in health policy and health education and back to its benefits viewed at a more individualistic level, this chapter will examine physical interfaces with history. Physical interaction might involve taking a day out to a historic monument or building, handling objects in a museum, using a museum or gallery as a community space, or getting on one's hands and knees and participating in an archaeological dig. These modes of engagement with the material world, where we walk into new spaces or literally turn historical artefacts over in our hands, bring us up close and personal to the past in a way that can feel more immediate, even confronting, than reading a history book on the sofa, researching in an archive or watching a historical documentary.

Lately, the therapeutic value of this physical engagement with history is demonstrated through the upswell of enthusiasm, in many governmental and clinical circles, for social prescribing. Yet, even when participatory engagement with historical objects and spaces is not formally prescribed by a doctor, the benefits of physical interactions with history are recognised more and more: they enhance people's sense of wellbeing, improve psychological and physical health, promote feelings of social inclusion and stimulate creativity.

Although the field of study which looks at the interrelationship between arts and heritage and health has blossomed over the past quarter of a century, the associations are not entirely new. In fact, the idea that art and galleries can have strong emotional effects on their visitors has a long history. One oft-cited early example is in the case of Stendhal who, when relating the details of his 1817 trip to Italy, declared that the emotional turmoil of seeing so much beauty had made him feel terribly unwell. Stendhal recollected in his writings how he had emerged from the doors of the exquisite Sante Croce Church in Florence with fluttering palpitations and a powerful feeling of faintness. Although occasional examples of fainting or becoming ill in the face of great art have been recorded since the nineteenth century, 'Stendhal syndrome' only became clinically categorised in 1979, when it was described by Italian psychiatrist Graziella Magherini who observed over a 100 similar cases among tourists in Florence. The central idea was that the beauty of art, artefacts and architecture could be so overwhelming that it could lead to feelings of unwellness in its observers. Although most of us are familiar with that feeling of almost swooning in reaction to great beauty, responses are usually not so severe; these days, Stendhal syndrome is rarely diagnosed. In fact, in diametrical opposition to the Stendhal principle, engaging with art and artefacts can inspire positive responses that feed into feelings of self-worth and wellness. Interaction with beauty or creativity is generally positioned as something which makes participants feel better, rather than worse.

In the chapter that follows 1 work from this generally accepted axiom that *heritage helps health*, presenting some of the good health outcomes linked to physical interaction with history. The most obvious avenue is the improvement of mental health (where interaction has been shown to elevate mood and self-esteem and reduce loneliness and isolation), but positive outcomes have also been identified in other areas – for example, enhancing experiences for people with neurological conditions, as exemplified in the positive results for dementia patients involved in museum health studies. Improvements in physical health (through the light exercise and reduced stress levels many of the interactions promote) have also been recorded, although this area is less frequently researched.

HOW CAN MUSEUMS AND HERITAGE INSTITUTIONS
HELP HEALTH?

The most obvious places where people can achieve hands-on or close-up interaction with history are museums and galleries, many of which are themselves housed within buildings of historical significance. Encompassing a range of establishments from small specialist museums to expansive national collections, most of these organisations are accessible with relatively little aid or effort. Some museums, admittedly mostly national collections, are free of entry charges and nearly all offer discounted admission tickets for children, students, the unwaged, the disabled and the retired. It may be surprising to some people to learn that a UK government review of museums in England estimated, fairly recently, that 55% of the UK population lived within walking distance of a museum or gallery (Mendoza, 2017, p. 20).[1]

Yet, despite museums and galleries being prominent, proximate and accessible, aside from a few (albeit growing number of) examples that I shall touch on later, the wellbeing potential of museums and galleries still remains largely under-explored. Even when museums or galleries host events targeted at health and wellbeing, these are often temporary or single initiatives. In short, although things are improving, there is still some way to go before health and wellbeing are routinely regarded as part of the core work of all heritage organisations. Furthermore, as pointed out some years ago, for museums to fully integrate health into their public offering, health and wellbeing need to be strategically embedded within the museum and heritage planning, design and evaluation (Chatterjee & Noble, 2016, p. 5).[2] This is not only socially expedient – making the most of our heritage institutions and capitalising on much-loved, accessible community spaces – it is also financially prudent in that it directs people away from already pressurised clinical health services.

Problems in positioning museums at the heart of sustained health engagement projects are not just evident on the side of the organisations, however. Many museums struggle to achieve their targets for visitor numbers, a situation which has been exacerbated by the exigencies of the COVID-19 pandemic. Even in 2019, before the onset of the pandemic, an Art Fund report (based on an online survey of just over 2,500 UK adults) concluded that although people were decidedly aware of the positive health and wellbeing effects of visits to museums and galleries, they rarely attended these places with any regularity. Despite knowing what was good for them in theory, people found that they struggled to find the time to fit visits into their routines. While 51% of people surveyed said that they would like to go to museums and galleries more often, it was striking that only 6% of respondents could claim that they regularly attended such institutions at least once a month. The reasons for this lack of take-up are complex and they vary between different demographic groups. While older people had more time available, their confidence to make visits was more likely to be influenced by physical or cognitive impairments, or social anxieties. In working-age people, the factors inhibiting regular visits tended to relate to lack of time and the persistent impacts of daily stressors and demands. Parents with school-aged children and full-time jobs, unsurprisingly, came out in the survey as experiencing the highest levels of stress, anxiety and time pressure. People aged 24–44, city-dwellers and women, reported being the most time-poor and stressed as they juggled the multiple challenges of their lives (Deuchar, 2019).[3]

Yet, even though the vast majority of people evidently do not find the time to visit sites of heritage and history, the benefits of heritage engagement seem hard to contest. Walking into these repositories of history, one can be transported 'away from it all', both chronologically (immersing oneself in a different time period) and aesthetically (through looking at past workmanship or artistry). Purposeful time out in museums and galleries, almost irrespective of the form they take, has been shown to be good for helping us to re-set our headspace and regain perspective and control. These history-orientated trips, which can be taken alone or with companions, give us new insights and learning, additional topics of conversation, opportunities for fun, as well as moments of calm and reflection.

These ideas are very much corroborated by Helen Chatterjee's work on the therapeutic potential of museums and art galleries. Such research studies have shown how heritage organisations can encourage exercise and social interaction, provide distraction in pain management, help to combat loneliness and social isolation (particularly in ageing populations and among those with mental health difficulties) and can be used as sites for advancing the cross-generational transfer of knowledge. The results can vary according to situational and personal circumstances, but the principal health effects collated by Camic and Chatterjee (2013)[4] remain pertinent today. Museum visits improve:

- Sense of connection and belonging.

- Human capital: using and improving skills.

- Optimism and hope.

- Moral values and beliefs.

- Identity capital and self-esteem.

- Emotional capital and resilience.

- Opportunity for success.

- Recognition of achievement.

- Support.

- Quiet, rest and sanctuary.

- Social capital and relationships.

- Meaningful pursuits.

- Safe and rich museum environment.

- Access to arts and culture.

In recent times, it is not just the provision of health-related services within heritage sites that have improved – so has the evaluation of their use. Helen Chatterjee has developed a measurement scale (the Museum Wellbeing Measures Toolkit) which allows museum professionals and clinicians to evaluate psychological or subjective wellbeing impacts and the effectiveness of both one-off activities and programmes of connected events. This model has been rolled out to many UK-based museums, allowing more organisational participants to take initiatives forward in their own institutions, tailored to their own specific interests (Thomson & Chatterjee, 2015).[5]

It is through these ever more sophisticated and measurable approaches that museums, galleries and exhibition spaces find themselves growing as community anchors. As well as providing venues for social gatherings or projects for learning in the community, they create spaces where people can reflect on their personal identity in predictable or unexpected ways. As remarked by Katherine Cotter:

> *When we enter a museum, we're entering it with an intention. We're entering this particular space that has unique art, architecture, and has unique things that we're going to be seeing whether it's an art museum or another form of museum or cultural institution .... We engage different mindsets and different cognitive processes. Once we get into the meat and potatoes of the museum visit, we see ourselves more concerned communally, thinking about how things are interrelated in the world more broadly. (cited by Crimmins, 2022)[6]*

Museums and galleries thus can be conceptualised as sites which transform history into action. History in these spaces is not theoretical, imagined through the pages of a book. Within museums and galleries, people can be brought together to discuss the subject – a process which expands intellectual understanding, but also deepens community social ties, improves social skills and reduces social anxieties. Several studies which can be accessed via the reference list at the end of Chapter 6 have enlarged current research understandings of the health benefits of engaging with these spaces. Some of these have charted the benefits for members of specific populations, such as socially displaced people (Chatterjee et al., 2020); young students (Rodéhn, 2020); children (Edeiken, 2012); people with chronic pain (Koebner et al., 2022); stroke rehabilitation patients (Morse, Thomson, Elsden, Rogers, & Chatterjee, 2022) and mental health patients (DeNil & Janssens, 2020). Of course, during the COVID-19 pandemic, new priorities also came to the fore, in terms of seeing museums as spaces of community connectivity (virtual and in-person) during a time where most people were living in comparative isolation (Mughal, Thomson, Daykin, & Chatterjee, 2022).

The benefits of drawing on these institutions, who act as custodians of history, are increasingly made plain by moves to put social prescribing at the heart of routine community medical provision. Social prescribing is the term used to describe the referral that a general practitioner makes to direct a patient to social activities for their health improvement, rather than (or alongside) pointing them towards medication or other physical or mental therapies. Although this book principally draws on examples within the UK context, it is worth noting that social prescribing programmes are widely implemented globally. Countries which regularly offer such provisions include the USA, China, South Korea, Japan, Singapore, Australia, New Zealand, Canada, Germany, Denmark, Sweden, Finland and Holland.

In the UK, social prescribing has occurred in some form since the early 1990s, but its use has accelerated since the 2010s. A study of 86 schemes (under the banner of 'Museums on Prescription', 2014–2017) which utilised social prescribing in central London and Kent, for example, reported increased 'self-esteem and confidence; improvement in mental wellbeing and positive mood; and reduction in anxiety, depression, and negative mood' in participants (Chatterjee, Camic, Lockyer, & Thomson, 2018, p. 97).[7] More recently, social prescribing has become formally embedded in UK government policy, notably in the most recent *NHS Long Term Plan* of 2019. Indicative of this new focus, the National Academy for Social Prescribing was launched in October 2019, a charity whose express aim is to standardise practices and improve training and awareness in the area. Since 2019, the Annual Social Prescribing Day has acted as a focal point to link local and national organisations and individuals involved in social prescribing, to raise awareness of its benefits.

We will now dig a little deeper into some of the specific ways that interacting within history-orientated settings can help our health. The literature on this topic is immense, so I touch only briefly on (a) the role of museums and exhibitions as sites of public health education, (b) object-focussed initiatives, (c) schemes and

events for dementia sufferers, the elderly and their carers, (d) the
potential of using archival collections for wellbeing and health, (e)
archaeology for health and wellbeing and, lastly, (f) the importance
of these material interactions for physical health.

How Can Going to a Museum Educate Us on Health?

Museums are of course sites for pursuing leisure but they are
also places from which public health education can be promoted
through historical examples, through permanent collections or special exhibitions. Although there are some very old medical history
museums, such as the Surgeons' Hall Museums (founded 1699) in
Edinburgh, Scotland, the extensive pathology collections within the
Musée Fragonard, France (founded 1766), the Berlin Museum of
Medical History at the Charité, Germany (1899) and the Dresden
Hygiene Museum (1911), to name a few prime examples, museums with health collections (and even those without them) did not
really begin to see themselves as partners in public health advocacy
until after the World War One. Even when the tide did slowly begin
to turn, permanent and temporary health-related displays in the
first half of the twentieth century tended to be straightforwardly
educative in focus. Information was almost always disseminated in
a top-down way and curators were less concerned with showcas-
ing actual experiences, or with encouraging debate, reflection or
even health improvements. Drawing a contrast between one of the
earliest health exhibits (at the American Museum of Health, 1939–
1940) and a very recent one ('Cancer Revolution', 2021–2022, at
the Science Museum, London) is illustrative here and shows how
the focus of curators has subtly, but significantly, changed over the
course of the last 100 years.

When the American Museum of Health opened to great media
attention at the World's Fair in New York in 1939, the highlight
of the exhibition was the 'Transparent Man', an impressive, large-
scale display which lit up the internal workings of the human body.
The exhibit was meant to be visual education at its best, and it
was viewed by more than 12 million visitors. However, as others
have argued since, the display's static nature put the onus of health
interpretation on the viewers so it was ultimately somewhat limited

in educative value (McLeary & Toon, 2012).[8] The emphasis for the visitor was on looking, and on receiving information (via recorded commentary which explained the functions of the various organs highlighted in turn). These descriptions were simple and straightforward and stopped short of being too directive. There was no room for discussing experience or subjective feelings, or the potentially differing points of view between doctors and patients.

Fast forward to the UK in 2021 and we see the much more complex curation of a health-orientated show. Rather than asking the public to make links through their own observations, exhibitions in recent years have been much more explicit in their intention to catalyse behaviour changes or raise public awareness. Examples are numerous, but I have singled out 'Cancer Revolution: Science, Innovation and Hope' which showed first at the Science and Industry Museum in Manchester (October 2021–March 2022) before moving to the Science Museum London (May 2022–January 2023). This exhibition, sponsored by Cancer Research UK, not only showcased the history of cancer prevention and its treatment, but also the experiences of clinicians, researchers, policymakers and patients. The express aim was to bring together experiences of cancer from the past with lived experiences today. As such, the curated material raised awareness of symptoms, methods of treatment and common ground in people's stories. One of the self-declared objectives of the exhibition, furthermore, was to instil hope. Visitors were also challenged to explore their diverse, perhaps even uncomfortable, reactions to the disease and its impacts.[9]

In many ways, the Cancer Revolution exhibition represents only the most recent stepping stone in a long lineage of health exhibits which have become progressively bolder and more socially interventionist in their public health objectives. A prominent early example in the UK was 'Exploring Living Memory', a project of the London History Workshop Centre, which came together in 1981 to encourage the development of reminiscence work throughout London. It culminated in an exhibition in 1984–1985 at London's Royal Festival Hall where displays were put together by various groups from schools and adult education colleges, pensioners' clubs and local history societies, patients in hospitals, community organisations and individuals. This curation 'from below', allowed the public to choose what was shown and to shape the direction of the exhibition.

Over the Atlantic, the drive to shape public health exhibitions as educative and hope-inspiring has also gained prominence. For example, in 2008, the Children's Museum of Manhattan partnered with the National Institutes of Health to produce an exhibition in response to growing concerns over childhood obesity in the USA. The aim of the show was to encourage children and their adult caregivers to pursue healthier eating behaviours. What was particularly innovative about this approach, however, was its emphasis on community involvement. To this end, a 'community feedback loop' enabled the museum to conduct needs assessments with community stakeholders, develop resources based on those assessments, implement them in the community and construct formal evaluations to assess their effectiveness (Ackerman, 2016).[10]

A common factor here is the devolution of some of the curatorial responsibilities. This has the advantage of giving ownership to the communities, which in turn can have knock-on positive effects on social inclusion. In the UK, a small-scale local example of this kind of engagement can be seen in an exhibition in 2015 by the Hampshire Cultural Trust which centred on the 200-year-old historic relationship between the British army and the Gurkhas, many of whom settled locally and are part of the local community. To foster greater cross-generational and cross-cultural awareness, the scheme encouraged young people between the ages of 12 and 18 to work with members of the local Nepali community to develop a photographic exhibition and an accompanying book. This involved many of the school-aged participants taking exhibition-quality photographs of the ex-Ghurkhas, interviewing them and deciding what elements of the history the public might be interested in discovering (https://www.hampshireculture.org.uk/social-impact/ gurkha-connection). As the promotional video on the project website attests, this was a really important project for many of the children involved, boosting their confidence, raising awareness of the histories of their community members and enfolding them in a series of interactivities that they might otherwise have assumed held no relevance for them.

Additional to these temporary exhibitions are the large permanent collections of health historical materials. Once again, the list is far too long to mention all, but several of these institutions have used their collections for opening dialogues about public health. Some prominent UK examples include: The Florence Nightingale Museum, London; The Hunterian Museum at the Royal College of Surgeons, London; The George Marshall Medical Museum, Worcester; the Wellcome Library collection, London; and the Thackray Museum of Medicine in Leeds. These specialist collections are also joined by the permanent galleries within the British Museum and the Science Museum London which showcase medical and health themes in their historical contexts.

Health historical exhibits are perhaps the most obvious medium via which educative public health interventions can be mobilised, but improving health does, of course, involve much more than improving health education. Museums and galleries – almost regardless of their thematic contents – are increasingly recognised as useful in other ways for the promotion of health and wellbeing. All hold historic objects and artefacts, all provide community spaces and all provide a break from familiar homes and working environments.

How Can Engaging with Historical Objects be Useful?

Objects are important material representations of history. Whether they are artefacts displayed in a museum cabinet and carefully curated, or personal family history objects carefully stored at the back of a drawer or in a box in the attic, material culture carries emotions and ideas of startling intensity. Increasingly, curators and museum educators are harnessing the power of their collections for building empathy, particularly through object-based learning experiences. Crow and Bowles (2018) have gone so far as to label museums as 'empathy engines': the objective to improve empathy specifically works because the objects offer a bridge between the new and unfamiliar and the handler's own experiences and points of view (p. 342).[11]

A number of initiatives within museums have used the handling of objects, or sometimes replica objects, to provide for tactile engagement and playful encounters as part of the museums' community outreach. As well as stimulating community cohesion, these sorts of events also spark curiosity, especially when the use of an object is initially unclear. Chatterjee, Vreeland and Noble found that object handling triggered two main responses. First, it encouraged people to talk about themselves and their ideas. Second, these activities revealed a hunger for learning more – acting more as a jumping-off point for further exploration than as an end in themselves. Both levels of response – which were sometimes experienced simultaneously – promoted positive feelings of wellbeing in people (Chatterjee, Vreeland, & Noble, 2009).[12] I would add to this point that object handling has the additional advantage of being inclusionary to those with hearing or sight loss. It is also an activity which is mentally accessible to those with long-term memory loss (as touched on in the section on dementia below).

Another example can be seen in the written evaluation of a community project conducted at the New Walk Museum and Art Gallery in Leicester, England. Here, school students were invited to handle 3,000-year-old Egyptian amulets. Certainly, the excitement aroused was partially borne of being *allowed* to touch something so ancient and authentic. The students' comments after the event pointed to the upbeat feelings inspired by this object interaction. A schoolgirl called Abby described the event as 'cool, it's like you're touching part of the past. You think maybe an Egyptian touched that at some point' (Dodd & Jones, 2014, p. 29).[13]

Yet, object handling needs not only to take place within the heritage site. The beauty of historical objects is their portability. If insurance constraints allow, artefacts can be brought into settings that customarily do not include them. Good outcomes have been observed, for example, when museum objects are brought into hospitals, care homes or support centres (Chatterjee & Noble, 2009).[14]

And it is not just handling which can be therapeutic. People might describe or otherwise interact with museum objects in a quasi-official capacity as a museum volunteer guide or volunteer researcher. Or individuals might use certain objects for inspiration to lead a creative practice (such as painting or document transcription) within a heritage space. Several important volunteering initiatives have been described in the 2018 report by the

National Alliance for Museums, Health & Wellbeing. Common responses from museum volunteer participants described increased confidence, improved social skills, lessening of anxieties and the comforting security of having a routine (Desmarais, Bedford, & Chatterjee, 2018).[15]

How Might Museum and Gallery Spaces Help Older Communities, Particularly Those with Dementia?

Museum object handling and other initiatives based in heritage institutions or in other settings (such as a museum or gallery resources brought into care homes) have proved remarkably successful for older people. Many of the elderly population live with physical frailty and/or disability and may also have cognitive impairment. It is not uncommon for older people, even those in good health, to feel socially redundant – often because individuals in the last quarter of their lives often start to feel that their social identities, previously caught up in busy professional or domestic roles, no longer exist or are no longer valued. Furthermore, in older populations, feelings of social isolation and loneliness can contribute to poorer wellbeing outcomes, creating states of mind that can further limit the likelihood of the person accessing opportunities for social interaction in the future.

Several programmes have been rolled out across the UK examining the better integration of social and cultural museum activities with the routine work of registered health and social care professionals. One such initiative in North East England is the Museum Health and Social Care Service (MHSCS) which provides a training resource for health and social care professionals. This resource, started in 2020, had the express aim to support practitioners delivering frontline health and social care to integrate heritage activities into their care plans. The initial results have been positive: elderly recipients of this scheme reported better self-esteem and improved wellbeing and therefore quality of life (Thompson et al., 2020).[16]

In dementia care, some research studies have recorded positive outcomes, especially in people who exhibit early or middle-stage dementia symptoms. Approaches vary. Some studies have found it beneficial to use objects with dementia sufferers to stimulate their personal memories and recollections of life experiences (Dudley, 2013; Froggett, Farrier, & Poursanidou, 2011).[17] In other studies, the preferred strategy was to use questions about the handled object, but not specifically probing for personal memories. Questions might include: What do you think this was used for? How could it have been used? What is it made of? When do you think it was produced? This latter approach has the benefit of being less likely to accidentally trigger any unhappy or traumatic memories (Camic, Hulbert, & Kimmel, 2019, p. 791).[18] The focus is on cultivating enjoyment in the present.

One of the oldest and most successful museum-led initiatives for dementia sufferers was at the Museum of Modern Art (MoMA) in New York: the 'Meet me at MoMa' project. This ran conference presentations and training workshops between 2007 and 2014 and involved the roll-out of a series of events and workshops specifically targeted at dementia patients and (quite originally for the time) their carers. The impact was measured via self-rating and observer-rating scales. In both cases, results were positive, showing better interaction and mood after discussing the artworks (Rosenburg, Parsa, Humble, & McGee, 2009).[19] This project was a departure from the model of handling artefacts and instead centred on viewing paintings to stimulate discussions and activities. The success of this initiative meant that it rapidly expanded, developing programme models and training and encouraging aligned museum professionals also to use their collections and spaces for their own engagement opportunities for the dementia community (https://www.moma.org/visit/accessibility/meetme/index.html). In Australia, the National Gallery now also holds art and dementia programmes (https://nga.gov.au/events/art-and-dementia-online/) and in the UK, a similar museum-led dementia awareness initiative can be found at the House of Memories Programme, National Museums Liverpool (https://www.liverpoolmuseums.org.uk/house-of-memories/about).

A notable feature of these schemes is that they include dementia carers, who often find themselves (and their psychological needs) overlooked when medical interventions prioritise the patient. The comfort provided by museum and heritage institution schemes can be transformational in recognising the challenges experienced by carers when a relative or close friend is given a diagnosis. The

House of Memories project in Liverpool uses moving video stories as a way of providing information and support to carers and
families of dementia sufferers. Similarly, the Birmingham Museums
Trust has run the Creative Carers Programme since 2016, offering
free art activities in a museum setting as a means of offering respite, outside the world of health and social care, to those caring for
someone with dementia.

HOW CAN ARCHIVAL COLLECTIONS BE USEFUL FOR HEALTH?

Visiting heritage sites— – whether for a casual stroll around the
collections or to participate in an object-handling event or community workshop – is not the only way in which health and wellbeing can benefit from museum holdings. The archival collections of
some organisations have also been used in targeted, often innovative, ways to promote a public health agenda and to improve community health. One of the best of these occurred in Nottingham at
the beginning of the 2010s when Nottingham City Museums and
Galleries used the extensive collections of the John Player & Sons
Archive in a secondary school project aiming to tackle the high
levels of smoking in the city. Working with Smokefree Nottingham
and the Public Health Development Manager of Nottingham City
Council, the museum service came up with a scheme to contribute to the city council's aim of reducing smoking prevalence to
the national average of 20%. The project that ensued, 'Live Today,
Think Tomorrow', involved piloting a set of resources for school
and youth groups that would address contemporary issues around
smoking by exploring archival materials, particularly those which
showed how cigarette advertising historically had glamourised
smoking or even associated it with better health (e.g. through sporting imagery). Project impact was captured by asking the young
people who took part to complete a response card: 69% of participants said that they had found out something 'new or unexpected'
about smoking through the activity sessions with archival material,
while 65% stated that the sessions had changed their mind about
smoking because the participants had learned more about the harm
it causes to health (Dodd & Jones, 2014, pp. 38–39).[20]

Another archival adventure designed to achieve improved health outcomes is the 'Change Minds' project based at Norfolk Heritage Centre, UK, and partnered with the arts-focussed mental health charity the Restoration Trust. This community research project focussed on two digitised nineteenth-century Norfolk County Asylum Case Books at the Norfolk Record Office and Norwich Millennium Library. Participants with mental health challenges were encouraged to learn conservation and document-handling skills, read the asylum archive case notes, participate in creative workshops, visit the old asylum and – if they wished – to record their own oral histories describing living with the consequences of mental health, for future generations (https://changeminds.org.uk/). The project proved to be popular and initiated discussions of lived experiences, comparing the past and the present in ways that helped people reflect on their own situations.

HOW CAN ARCHAEOLOGY BE USEFUL FOR HEALTH AND WELLBEING?

Although the value of museums and galleries for health and wellbeing has been simmering for several decades, it is more recently that the health benefits of *physically doing* history, via community archaeology projects, have been recognised.

A project that was transformational in moving attention to the therapeutic value of archaeology was Operation Nightingale, a venture that originated from an unlikely source – The UK Ministry of Defence. It started in 2011 in conjunction with Wessex Archaeology, using archaeological activities as a means of aiding the recovery, and skill development, of service personnel injured in recent conflicts, particularly in Afghanistan (https://www. wessexarch.co.uk/our-work/operation-nightingale). During the first phase of the project, a Bronze Age burial mound and Saxon cemetery were excavated at Barrow Clump in the Salisbury Plain training area. Participants found several Saxon burial graves, as well as some exciting jewellery, warfare and household objects. Since its start, Operation Nightingale has involved hundreds of military personnel in its projects which now run in several UK locations as well as overseas. Its methods have become well-established as an efficacious way to reintegrate ex-service people, especially the wounded, into civilian life.

Building on this highly successful project, several other initiatives have emerged. One such project, set up in 2015 also with military personnel in mind, is Breaking Ground Heritage. This organisation encourages participation in projects which use heritage generally, but archaeology specifically, as a recovery pathway. Partnerships with several UK-based educational institutions and professional organisations offer opportunities for veterans to study further or to gain experience within commercial archaeology. A testimonial by a former member of the Royal Tank Regiment provides a moving tribute to the scheme:

> *Being part of the team at Bullecourt was amazing, as someone with a keen interest in History, its real hands-on experience and a chance to get more in depth in our History that's evolved over the years. And actually finding parts of a first war tank and being able to help preserve it for future generation and my own regiments history made is so worthwhile.*
>
> *Also, it was chance to put my own injuries aside and try forget the barriers I have to live with, for which Breaking Ground Heritage as been able to do while taking part in this dig, and also has made me overcome barriers both physically and mentally as well.*[21]

Others attest to the way the project has helped them overcome PTSD or depression. For many who have served in the forces, return to civilian life is often very difficult, not only because of the traumas witnessed while serving, but also because their identity has become bound up for so long in their military role. Especially in the current context of rising military suicides, projects such as this are vital for helping veterans cope with traumatic memories and social dislocation.

These kinds of archaeology – focussed projects achieve many of the therapeutic benefits that have been identified in museum and gallery – based health projects. Participating in a dig, or joining a metal detector enthusiasts' group, builds social inclusion, increases confidence and creates a shared group purpose that can be reaffirming to individuals who, for a variety of reasons, might otherwise find it difficult to socially integrate. However, in addition to these positive outcomes, another therapeutic theme emerges out of the archaeological engagement – connectivity to the land.

At its simplest, participating in an excavation or going out with a metal detector involves being outside, close to earth and vegetation, and sometimes braving the elements. These things in and of themselves are widely regarded as important for improving health and wellbeing. The participants themselves often think of these hobbies as a form of self-therapy, a way to get them out and about and to relax and re-focus away from their usual stresses and strains. A 2020 study in Denmark showed that over 70% of survey participants involved with metal detecting felt that the activity boosted their mood. Furthermore, this mood elevation fed directly into improved mental and physical wellbeing. Precisely because the activity was 'hands-on', it captured – according to one participant – 'the thrill of history', the sense of excitement evoked through participating in 'real' archaeological research, even if only as a hobbyist (Dobat, Dobat, & Schmidt, 2022, pp. 150, 156).[22] More details connected to this initiative appear as the case study at the end of this chapter.

But for many individuals, the therapeutic benefit is wider than feeling better for being outdoors in nature: they value the proximity such participatory work encourages with the broader environmental agenda. The work involves people with issues 'bigger' than themselves. They actively use history as a means of improving the future, through better understanding our relationship with, and sometimes preserving, the landscapes in which we live.

A focus on the health benefits of connectivity with the land might also in some circumstances have broader socio-political dimensions. There are several projects which have sought to decolonise archaeology and have used their discipline to reach, and return agency to, indigenous communities. For example, in South Australia, a large-scale archaeological initiative has worked with the Ngadjuri people. Although the project, which commenced in 1998, was initially led by academic researchers, ultimately it passed leadership over to the Ngadjuri themselves. This Aboriginal group had been disposed of their land since the British colonisation of Australia in the 1830s. Even in cases where they had been allowed to live on their ancestorial land, they had become increasingly dislocated from their traditional pasts through intrusive foreign incursions. In this project, voluntary involvement in archaeological excavations became a way for Ngadjuri to reconnect with their land and self-determine their cultural heritage. Although the damage of colonisation had been done, project participation nevertheless marked a step towards repairing some of the community's social, economic and emotional connectivity with their revered ancestors. The opportunity to map their own history revealed to new Ngadjuri generations their rich artistic-cultural heritage. It also provided information on the people's demographic movements over time, as well as insights into their historic quotidian practices (farming, subsistence and domestic duties). This information not only serves to help to rewrite a more accurate history of Australia but also feeds into conservation projects that look to protect the rights and heritage of indigenous people. Furthermore, the wellbeing outcomes for the Ngadjuri people themselves were notable, perhaps even more so because they represent a community where wellbeing is inseparably bound up in group kinship models and spiritual connectivity to the land. For them, as expressed by the project's Ngadjuri lead, Vincent Copley, archaeology was a means of reasserting traditional authority, having their human rights recognised, acknowledging their cultural diversity and returning agency and self-determination to a community that had been dispossessed (Smith, Copley, Lower, Kotaba, & Jackson, 2022).[23]

In this example, archaeology has been used to enhance cultural identity and thereby goes some small way to restoring the dignity of people who have been exploited in history. Although archaeological endeavour is clearly not the only way to achieve these ends, in this instance, the activities seemed particularly well suited to the communities involved, precisely because of their spiritual relationship with their lands. Archaeology gave participants a culturally relevant way to further explore their identities. It provided participants with a new tool to develop historical consciousness, bringing the additional social benefit of feeding into the development and continuation of cultural identity in the youth community members.

ARE THERE PHYSICAL BENEFITS AS WELL AS PSYCHOLOGICAL ONES?

Reflecting the majority of the available literature on the topic, most of this chapter has focussed on heritage-related interactions as a means of enhancing mental health, life satisfaction and well-being. However, it should not be forgotten that museums and archaeological digs can also be seen as places to promote better physical health. An in-person visit to a heritage site almost always involves some physical movement and discourages sedentary behaviours. Even better, participating in an excavation, or combing an area for artefacts with a metal detector, can involve walking for several hours. Whether heritage-related exercise is strenuous or very light, it generally brings the benefit of physical motion and activity. At its very simplest, in museum and gallery settings, people are encouraged to walk from room to room. Whereas an outside activity might be bracing, for the less physically fit a museum or gallery can offer a safe space to gently exercise. Heritage institutions commonly provide warm and comforting environments and usually have seating points where the elderly and infirm can rest.

As one witty blogger wryly noted on her personal website, she always lost weight on holiday because of what she called 'The Museum Diet'. Basically, walking around museums can take a lot of energy! The same blogger estimated that to go around the Vatican was a nine-mile walk, the Victoria and Albert Museum a seven-mile walk, The Louvre, eight miles and the Smithsonian nearly 10 miles (Tammy Tour Guide, 2014).[24] In fact, many museums and galleries have realised that their buildings provide ample space to host exercise classes. To this end, both the Metropolitan Museum of Art and MoMa in New York offer group workout sessions set to disco music in front of art masterpieces.

In 2016, the Kunsthaus in Graz, Austria, even showcased a good-humored project developed by artist Aldo Giannotti, which explored the use of the museum as a gym for mind and body using only existing infrastructural features.[25] Free entry was offered to all those attending in sports gear. Although this was a temporary exhibition, specifically asking visitors to use the gallery to exercise, some heritage institutions use their capacious rooms for yoga and Pilates sessions on an ongoing basis. These new and imaginative ways of thinking about cultural spaces as places which can improve physical health represent a shift from traditional notions of museums and galleries as primarily highbrow intellectual sites.

Other researchers have identified added physiological benefits of museum and gallery visits, such as stress reduction as evidenced by the normalisation of salivary cortisol levels (Clow & Fredhoi, 2006).[26] As researcher Katherine Cotter has argued:

if you just go for half an hour to an art museum and measure people's cortisol levels before they go in, after half an hour it shows the kind of recovery time [normally] equivalent to a few hours. (cited by Crimmins, 2022)[27]

These findings build on other work which suggests that art gallery visits lower blood pressure and stress (Mastandrea et al., 2018).[28]

A study undertaken at the Montreal Museum of Fine Arts found that community attendees (usually older people) at their 'Thursdays at the Museum' programme experienced not only improved wellbeing but also physical benefits including healthier heart rates, higher step counts and better sleep patterns (Beauchet et al., 2020).[29] Similarly, hands-on examinations of objects and artefacts can help to improve coordination and motor skills as part of physical therapeutic regimes.

In some instances, it can be the *escape* that a visit to a gallery or heritage site symbolises which is the most important factor. Although most of the studies concerned with the health benefits of heritage visits talk about the reinforcement of community networks to tackle social isolation and loneliness, escapism can also be a way to help people feel better about themselves. Sometimes, immersing oneself in looking at objects outside of one's daily experience can be a means of forgetting daily struggles, bringing a sense of respite that can be especially helpful for those living with chronic conditions or daily pain. In these cases, the ability to detach from one's difficulties, even if only temporarily, can be of huge importance.

* * *

We have seen that physical cultural participation in history can take many forms: ranging from high-level discussions of artefacts, to wandering around an installation on a rainy afternoon, to attending a more playful workshop using replica objects or costumes, to participating in a community archaeological dig. Regardless of form, participation can be harnessed to do valuable health work, both preventative and remedial. By coming up close to our history, through the relics and cultural production which fortunately have survived the vagaries of time, we raise our gaze and engage with our current moment, relative to the moments that are behind us. Touching history might not be a medical treatment or a cure in the same way that taking a tablet might be, but as so many studies attest, visiting museums and galleries improves most people's sense of worth and feelings of life satisfaction. It boosts self-esteem and self-confidence, improves sociability, elevates mood, increases cognitive functioning and positively impacts cardiovascular and muscular health and bodily chemical balances.

Furthermore, engagement with history in this way helps us, as citizens, to make connections that are important for positioning ourselves and anchoring our lives. Thinking about our forebears can be a useful way not only to ponder ourselves but also to remind us of our universality. As such, museums and galleries should be seen as important sites for the recovery and restoration of knowledge of ourselves and the communities and nations to which we belong. They are particularly valuable as they perform the seemingly contradictory work of increasing people's sense of autonomy while also making them feel more connected to their communities. Both of these forces have been shown to improve health and wellbeing.

CASE STUDY 3: SEARCHING FOR ARCHAEOLOGICAL ARTEFACTS, FINDING PATHS TO WELLBEING: HOW HOBBY ARCHAEOLOGY AND METAL DETECTORS MAY IMPROVE QUALITY OF LIFE

ANDRES S. DOBAT AND AJA SMITH

Description of Project

Sometimes I wake from a dream and don't know whether I am with my wife or in Iraq …. And then I know I need to go out, searching with the detector ….

Reflections such as this one which directly relates archaeological metal detecting to a kind of self-therapy are common among participants in the Danish *Vetektor Buddy Program*. In this programme, veterans are provisioned with the necessary technical gear and paired with experienced metal detectorists who act as mentors introducing them to the hobby. While only some of the veterans are clinically diagnosed, they all suffer from mental health issues related to their military deployments. They describe how archaeological metal detecting has become a tool to improve their mental health and quality of life.

It is not only in Denmark that the activity of searching for archaeological artefacts with a metal detector has been associated with improved mental health and wellbeing. Nor is the perception of such positive effects of the hobby limited to people with mental health problems, veterans or otherwise. In fact, searching for archaeological artefacts with a metal detector has developed into a popular leisure activity across Europe, and the idea of metal detecting as contributing positively to both mental health and general wellbeing is highlighted in conversations among members of metal detector communities and on social media.

While the professional heritage sector, museums and archaeologists tend to focus on the nature of the produced archaeological artefacts be they Roman brooches, medieval coins or material traces of more recent conflicts, the qualities which the metal detectorists themselves associate with their hobby seem to branch into a much broader territory. But what is it about the activity of metal detecting that makes both people with, and without, mental health issues alike experience such positive effects of the hobby? And what role do the search for artefacts and their link to history and national identity play in this experience? Focussing on detectorists' experiences of betterment, this case study highlights how archaeological metal detecting allows the individual a sense of self-efficacy, access to a community and a connection to a greater historical purpose.

Methodology

The findings are based on two online surveys with metal detector users in the UK and Denmark, and two qualitative interviews with veterans involved in the Danish *Vetektor Buddy Program*:

- In 2018, we conducted an online questionnaire aimed specifically at UK Armed Forces veterans and metal detector users with either undiagnosed or diagnosed mental health problems (Dobat, Wood, Jensen, Schmidt, & Dobat, 2020).[30] The survey focussed on questions regarding the effect participants perceived metal detection had on their health, wellbeing and diagnosed specific symptoms.

- In spring 2020, during the worldwide COVID-19 lockdown, we conducted a follow-up study among Danish metal detector users in which just under a quarter of the participants reported suffering or having suffered from mental issues (Dobat & Dobat, 2020).[31] The survey focussed on the perceived effect of metal detection on health and wellbeing and specifically in relation to general stress and anxiety caused by the COVID-19 situation and related measures.

- In 2022, two interviews were conducted with veterans suffering from PTSD. The veterans were participants in the *Vetektor Buddy Program* and had at the time of the interviews been paired with a mentor from a regional metal detector association. Detecting missions were either conducted alone or with a mentor but were always in an area where the mentor had secured the relevant permissions.

Findings

In this case study, we focus on detectorists' own perception and experience of the effects of their hobby and highlight three central factors; the activity of walking with a detector in nature; the sense of independence it by way of its informal nature grants; and the connection to a community and national history it fosters. While the study does not provide evidence of the effect of archaeological metal detecting in a clinical medical sense, these key findings resonate with clinically recognised pathways for enhancing mental health; physical exercise and mindfulness, time spent outdoors, connection to others and to purposes beyond oneself (see e.g. UK National Health Services, 2022).[32]

Walking in Nature: The very practice of walking with a metal detector is described as bringing participants to an almost meditative state. Detectorists often find themselves walking for hours on end, eyes fixed on the detector's digital display, the ground and the detector's search coil, attention fully captivated, the sensory system relaxed but attuned, the kinesthetic rhythm of the walk and uniform motions with the detector all contribute to general relaxation and easing of stress. Many participants link the relaxing quality of the hobby of metal detecting directly to being in nature; it is not least the nature of the hobby as an outdoor activity that is considered to impact positively on practitioners' sense of wellbeing. Yet, the activity in itself involves not only a mindful presence in nature but also a degree of physical exercise which all participants found positively impactful to their wellbeing.

Informality and Independence: In contrast to the medical monitoring involved in formal mental health programmes and the way most community archaeology projects are dependent on limited financial funding and the politics of private and public host institutions, metal detectorists remain largely autonomous and independent actors with little need for professional facilitation and guidance. The hobby can be practiced legally by anyone, at any time and anywhere, with appropriate permissions. Practitioners find such informality and independence crucial; whether they battle mental health problems or simply enjoy the positive effects of their hobby, they feel empowered to independently take charge of their own health and wellbeing.

Connection to Community and History: While the activity grants practitioners a high degree of independence, the hobby is not exclusively a solitary activity. In fact, archaeological metal detecting gives detectorists access to a casual community, where verbal interaction with others is optional and often minimal. The hobby transpires in a non-compulsory social arena, where detectorists remain in control of the extent of their social engagement and regardless form part of a community. Unsurprisingly, for many, the appeal of the hobby originates from its close ties to historical events; it is experienced as endowed with the thrilling qualities of global and national history, evoking a sense of excitement, adventure and even magic. Such links with history and not least national identity are crucial for participants' experience of the greater significance of their hobby. As they experience the success of finding artefacts of archaeological value, since the recognition from fellow detectorists and the public, and feel they contribute to a greater cause beyond themselves, they report an enhanced sense of self-esteem and wellbeing.

Suggested Future Research

Over the past years, metal detecting as a practice that enhances wellbeing has become an integral element of several community archaeology initiatives; for example, the US American Veterans Archaeology programme (https://americanveteransarchaeology. org/) or the research project and charity organisation Waterloo Uncovered (https://waterloouncovered.com/about/). Such initiatives' value lies in their dual function as classic and applied research; uncovering archaeological discoveries and enhancing participants' mental health.

At Aarhus University, we are in the process of upscaling the existing *Vetektor Buddy Program* to further deploy and explore the special quality of metal detecting as a potential source of wellbeing and mental health. Our aim is not simply to integrate a mental health initiative in archaeological research, but to also research the impact of such an initiative and on this basis to develop prototypes for how archaeology along with the heritage sector may support the mitigation of mental health issues and rehabilitation.

NOTES

1. Mendoza, N. (2017). *The Mendoza review: An independent review of museums in England*. Department for Digital, Culture, Media and Sport. Retrieved from https://www.gov.uk/government/publications/the-mendoza-review-an-independent-review-of-museums-in-england.

2. Chatterjee, H., & Noble, G. (2016). *Museums, health and well-being*. London: Routledge.

3. Deuchar, S. (2019). *Calm and collected, museums and galleries: The UK's untapped wellbeing resource*. London: The Art Fund.

4. Camic, P. M., & Chatterjee, H. J. (2013). Museums and art galleries as partners for public health interventions. *Perspectives in Public Health*, *133*(1), 66–71. https://doi.org/10.1177/1757913912468523.

5. Thomson, L. J., & Chatterjee, H. J. (2015). Measuring the impact of museum activities on well-being: Developing the museum well-being measures toolkit. *Museum Management and Curatorship*, *30*(1), 44–62. https://doi.org/10.1080/09647775.2015.1008390.

6. Crimmins, P. (2022, June 14). *Why visiting a museum is good for your health*. WITF News. Retrieved from https://www.witf.org/2022/06/14/why-visiting-a-museum-is-good-for-your-health/.

7. Chatterjee, H. J., Camic, P. M., Lockyer, B., & Thomson, L. J. M. (2018). Non-clinical community interventions: A systematised review of social prescribing schemes. *Arts & Health*, *10*(2), 97–123. https://doi.org/10.1080/17533015.2017.1334002.

8. McLeary, E., & Toon, E. (2012). "Here man learns about himself": Visual education and the rise and fall of the American Museum of Health. *American Journal of Public Health*, *102*(7), e27–e36. http://dx.doi.org/10.2105/AJPH.2011.300560.

9. Science Museum. (2022). *Cancer revolution: Science innovation and hope* (past exhibition). Retrieved from https://www.sciencemuseum.org. uk/what-was-on/cancer-revolution-science-innovation-and-hope.

10. Ackerman, A. (2016). Museums and health: A case study of research and practice at the Children's Museum of Manhattan. *Journal of Museum Education*, 41(2), 82–90. https://doi.org/10.1080/10598650.2016.1169727.

11. Crow, W., & Bowles, D. (2018). Empathy and analogy in museum education. *Journal of Museum Education*, 43(4), 342–348. https://doi.org/ 10.1080/10598650.2018.1529904.

12. Chatterjee, H., Vreeland, S., & Noble, G. (2009). Museopathy: Exploring the healing potential of handling museum objects. *Museum and Society*, 7(3), 164–177. https://discovery.ucl.ac.uk/id/eprint/1309194.

13. Dodd, J., & Jones, C. (2014). *Mind, body, spirit: How museums impact health and wellbeing*. Leicester: Research Centre for Museums and Galleries.

14. Chatterjee, H. J., & Noble, G. (2009). Object therapy: A student-selected component exploring the potential of museum object handling as an enrichment activity for patients in hospital. *Global Journal of Health Sciences*, 1(2), 42–49. http://dx.doi.org/10.5539/gjhs.v1n2p42.

15. Desmarais, S., Bedford, L., & Chatterjee, H. J. (2018). *Museums as spaces for wellbeing: A second report from the National Alliance for Museums, Health and Wellbeing*. https://museumsan dwellbeingalliance.files.wordpress.com/2018/04/mus eums-as-spaces-for-wellbeing-a-second-report.pdf.

16. Thompson, J., Brown, Z., Baker, K., Naisby, J., Mitchell, S., Dodds, C., … Collins, T. (2020). Development of the 'Museum Health and Social Care Service' to promote the use of arts and cultural activities by health and social care professionals caring for older people. *Educational Gerontology*, 46(8), 452–460. https://doi.org/10.1080/03601277.2020.1 770469.

17. Dudley, S. H. (2013). Museum materialities: Objects, sense and feeling. In S. H. Dudley (Ed.), *Museum materialities* (pp. 21–38). Routledge; Froggett, L., Farrier, A., & Poursanidou, K. (2011). *Who cares? Museums, health and wellbeing research project: A study of the*

Renaissance Northwest Programme. Preston: University of Central Lancashire.

18. Camic, P. M., Hulbert, S., & Kimmel, J. (2019). Museum object handling: A health-promoting community-based activity for dementia care. *Journal of Health Psychology*, 24(6), 787–798. https://doi.org/10.1177/1359105316685899.

19. Rosenberg, F., Parsa, A., Humble, L., & McGee, C. (2009). *Meet me: Making art accessible to people with dementia*. New York, NY: Museum of Modern Art.

20. Dodd, J., & Jones, C. (2014). *Mind, body, spirit: How museums impact health and wellbeing*. Leicester: Centre for Museums and Galleries.

21. Peter Cosgrove, Testimonial on breaking ground heritage. Retrieved from https://breakinggroundheritage.org.uk/about-1/. Accessed on December 30, 2022.

22. Dobat, A. S., Dobat, A. S., & Schmidt, S. (2022). Archaeology as "self-therapy": Case studies of metal detecting communities in Britain and Denmark. In P. Everill & K. Burnell (Eds.), *Archaeology, heritage, and wellbeing* (145–161). London: Routledge.

23. Smith, C., Copley, V., Lower, K., Kotaba, A., & Jackson, G. (2022). Using archaeology to strengthen Indigenous social, emotional, and economic wellbeing. In P. Everill & K. Burnell (Eds.), *Archaeology, heritage, and wellbeing* (pp. 119–144). London: Routledge.

24. Tammy Tour Guide. (2014, December 31). *The Museum Diet: How to lose weight on holiday*. Retrieved from https://tammytourguide.wordpress.com/2014/05/19/the-museum-diet-and-how-to-lose-weight-on-holiday/.

25. Kunsthaus, G. (2016). *The Museum as a gym: Fitness trail at the Kunsthaus Graz*. A Project by Aldo Giannotti. Retrieved from https://www.museum-joanneum.at/en/kunsthaus-graz/exhibitions/art-projects/temporary-projects/events/event/5130/the-museum-as-a-gym-3. Accessed from December 20, 2022.

26. Clow, A., & Fredhoi, C. (2006). Normalisation of salivary cortisol levels and self-report stress by a brief lunchtime visit to an art gallery by London City workers. *Journal of Holistic Healthcare*, 3(2), 29–32.

27. Crimmins, P. (2022, June 14). *Why visiting a museum is good for your health*. *WITF News*. Retrieved from https://www.witf.org/2022/06/1 4/why-visiting-a-museum-is-good-for-your-health/.

28. Mastandrea, S., Maricchiolo, F., Carrus, G., Giovannelli, I., Giuliani, V., & Berardi, B. (2018). Visits to figurative art museums may lower blood pressure and stress. *Arts & Health*, *11*(2), 123–132. https://doi.org/ 10.1080/17533015.2018.1443953.

29. Beauchet, O., Cooper-Brown, L., Hayashi, Y., Galery, K., Vilcocq, C., & Bastien, T. (2020). Effects of "Thursdays at the Museum" at the Montreal Museum of Fine Arts on the mental and physical health of older community dwellers: The art-health randomized clinical trial protocol. *Trials*, *21*(1), 1–12. https://doi.org/10.1186/s13063-020-04625-3.

30. Dobat, A. S., Wood, S. O., Jensen, B. S., Schmidt, S., & Dobat, A. S. (2020). "I now look forward to the future, by finding things from our past …" Exploring the potential of metal detector archaeology as a source of well-being and happiness for British Armed Forces veterans with mental health impairments. *International Journal of Heritage Studies*, *26*(4), 370–386. https://doi.org/10.1080/13527258.2019.1639069.

31. Dobat, A. S., & Dobat, A.S. (2020). Arkæologi som terapi: Metaldetektor hobbyen og mental sundhed i Danmark. *Arkæologisk Forum*, *43*, 11–24. http://www.archaeology.dk/17011/Nr.%2043%20-%202020.

32. UK National Health Service. (2022). Retrieved from https://www.nhs.uk/mental-health/self-help/guides-tools-and-activities/five-steps-to-mental-wellbeing/.

5

THE CHALLENGES AND
OPPORTUNITIES OF SUCCESSFUL
ENGAGEMENT WITH HISTORY

As the main part of this book has been devoted to extolling the benefits of history in the promotion of health and wellbeing, this chapter moves the focus to some of the challenges. Identifying these challenges is certainly not intended to put people off, but rather to highlight some potential hurdles so that participants and practitioners can anticipate them better. I prefer to think of this as awareness raising rather than a warning red light which might deter people. Outcomes are necessarily so personal that the unexpected might occur at any time. Equally, carefully anticipated problems simply might not arise.

In the second half of this chapter, I re-visit oral history as a topic because I believe oral history collections and archives are an important and oft-overlooked 'way in' to thinking about synergies between history and health. Oral history does unique work in capturing voices of lived experience, transporting complex subjectivities over time for successive generations. Furthermore, oral history's distinctively personal quality – allowing us to listen to people's thoughts first-hand – gives listeners unusually intimate access to the past. Hearing about these former health encounters can provide solace and comfort for those living today with health conditions. Although I have discussed in Chapter 2, the therapeutic benefits of being an oral history participant – whether as an inter-viewer or interviewee – my return to the subject here is to point readers in the direction of some of the most important oral his-tory collections. Although there are many steps people can take to mobilise history for health, these collections deserve special men-tion because they provide some of the most accessible and power-ful resources available to support individuals and their carers on their history and health journeys.

COMMON CHALLENGES TO SUCCESSFUL ENGAGEMENT WITH HISTORY FOR HEALTH

The following list of challenges is not definitive but draws out some of the key areas that might prove sticky for those thinking expan-sively about the ways history can help health. Many of the ideas have been alluded to in previous chapters, but here I specifically list key issues that patients, practitioners and carers can usefully reflect on.

History Is Not a Tool of Precedent to Apply Directly onto the Present

All too often people can be heard making casual reference to the importance of learning from the 'lessons' of history. Sadly, we rarely do. In fact, the hallmark of a good historian is to understand that no two contexts are ever exactly the same and, therefore, while we can see similarities in past trajectories which might guide our future behaviours, to use history with integrity one must be careful not to imbue past events with the character of a blueprint for the future. At its simplest, this means that history cannot fully work as a precedent because the system of social references that made something happen in the first instance can never be fully recreated. To take the hypothetical example of a diary of a cancer sufferer from 1950, a modern person with cancer might read this historic source with great interest, feeling an intense sense of connection with the historical subject's experiences and emotions. This con-nectivity might be useful because it helps the modern patient feel less alone and seems to underscore the universality of certain feelings (perhaps helplessness, perhaps unfairness, perhaps anger) or convey how common certain physiological health experiences might be. Yet, having cancer in 1950 was very different from having cancer today. This difference should be measured, not only in terms of available diagnostic technologies and treatments but also in terms of the world view which existed around the 1950s patient and their care team. How to *be* a cancer patient was different then to how it is now. Cancer was spoken about in subtly dissimilar ways, and a diagnosis was differently experienced, socially, politically and economically. The age, race and gender of the patient would have been personally embodied, and externally viewed, relational to the social mores of the time. Furthermore, no two people are alike. One person's experiences will never be precisely the same as another's. Historic source material might guide or inspire modern cancer patients, but ultimately these reference points cannot reliably predict how an individual will idiosyncratically react to a cancer diagnosis or will respond to treatments, even if several factors appear identical on the surface.

However, even if history cannot provide direct lessons and templates, it can offer valuable insights into possible alternatives, an assessment of which can empower consumers to critically examine their present situations and imagine a range of scenarios. We do history best when we realise that the past actors lived in a world different from our own, stimulated by social, political and cultural factors we might, or might not, recognise. I do not believe that acknowledging these contingencies should take away from the feelings of empathy and community that engagement with history elicits.

Be Careful That Our Modern Subjectivities Do Not Blind Us

Another challenge of history is that we sometimes, understandably, want to curate the past to say what we want it to say for our current circumstances. People are particularly susceptible to this hazard when they feel unwell, or when they are deeply involved in caring for someone who is unwell. If they are looking for stories of hope or inspiration, people might become so intent on having their needs validated by history that they may be blindsided into foregrounding one narrative ahead of another. In these cases, people consciously or subconsciously seek out stories that support their position, perhaps over-emphasising the contention that they want to have validated. At its worst, this urge can be so overwhelming that the adventurer into history might go so far as to ignore historical evidence that does not support their personal research agenda.

This is difficult terrain to navigate. While accepting that it is wrong to manipulate history to our modern ends, it is also vital to acknowledge that a good historian knows that truly objective history is impossible. We are all coloured by our life histories and our own social and political contexts when we read and write history. The key then is to get the balance right. The inescapability of some degree of subjectivity can be acknowledged, while at the same time, modern researchers need to be careful not to wistfully put words into our forebears' mouths or ascribe to them certain thoughts or agency that cannot be evidenced.

Historians can never know for sure if they have uncovered the 'true' story. History, when studied as an academic discipline, is about presenting options. Historical articles and books work to offer new interpretations, some of which may stand for a long time and some of which may be overturned or discredited quite quickly. The upshot of accepting that we will never really know precisely how things happened, or precisely what was in any historical actor's mind, means that all historical accounts are ultimately contestable, so long as persuasive evidence is presented. What's more, one historian might read the same source very differently to another. Rather than such ambiguity is an inherent weakness of the discipline, this can be its strength. A good historian will look at a range of primary and secondary evidence and offer their interpretation. History as a discipline, rather than seeking to provide definitive answers, intrinsically embraces uncertainty. This approach can be particularly helpful to those who are unwell. History allows its consumers to survey a wide range of possible outcomes and responses, but at the same time offers no certainty as to what our own outcome might be. This critical perspective can be liberating when hope sits at its centre.

Public History Is Curated

Challenges of historical subjectivity should also be considered in the context of public history. In Chapter 4, we spoke about the educative value of museums and galleries, particularly in terms of presenting public health messages in easily digestible ways to large audiences. Yet, of course, all museum education, including health education, is not neutral. Museums and heritage sites present selective and heavily curated versions of events. Collections of exhibits are built upon socially and politically informed selection decisions, budgetary limitations and space factors.

As recent research has shown, even when museums or exhibitions aim to showcase health topics in a dialogical and facilitative way, there can be an inbuilt instrumentalism within the goals of health promotion which can seem prescriptive and authoritative. This was eloquently described by Bønnelycke Grabowski, Christensen, Bentsen, and Jespersen (2021):

> [H]ealth-promoting exhibitions tend to reproduce normative and authoritative health education that defines health in specific ways and seeks to guide visitors in certain, predefined directions; a move that goes against the ideals of museums and science centres to provide open-ended and dialogic learning opportunities. (p. 288)[1]

Another issue which should be anticipated is the fact that curators cannot control how audiences will react to the displays. This can be both a hazard and a boon. An installation that is designed to educate and stimulate, might instead upset some viewers. The detailed presentation of the history of a certain health condition might be hugely informative for some people, but distressing and regressively triggering for others. Similarly, a historical investigation that is fascinating and psychologically supportive for one visitor, might awaken cross-generational trauma in another.

History Has Been Exclusionary

Aligned to the need to be aware of the power of curatorial authority, there is the need to be critically attuned to historical silences.

Even when analysing how people lived in the past, through the documents or artefacts which remain, we should pause and think about those who left behind little or no source material. Historical archives prioritise the voices of the literate and powerful. Bureaucracies leave detailed historical traces, whereas humble everyday lives rarely do. Transposed to a health historical context, this means that doctors and surgeons have left more source material than sufferers, patients or informal carers. It is much easier to learn about treatments and therapies from a top-down perspective than it is to access patient experiences. Even when those experiences were recorded in the past, they were usually refracted through the pen of the physician preparing the case note.

In historical records, the health experiences of women, the disabled and people of colour are less frequently documented than the work of public health administrators, powerful social reformers or the experiences of educated white men. This is not to say that the under-represented groups have left absolutely no trace in the archive, but critical historians should be keenly aware that much archival material represents merely one perspective within a much broader story. Furthermore, while in some cases source material never existed, in others it has been destroyed through historic decisions over archiving processes. In the past, for example, it might not have been anticipated that future generations would want to look at a 'mundane' diary or would deem the correspondence of a servant as worthy of keeping as the letters of a master.

In recent times, oral history and the popularity of the personal health memoir have expanded health information source bases, recording a wider range of experiences and reactions to health and wellbeing. However, some diseases and conditions are more frequently written about than others. While it is commonplace now to read an addiction recovery memoir or a cancer memoir, it is much harder (for example) to find accounts of sexually transmitted diseases or to hear about the everyday struggles of those with disfigurements and disabilities. It is also rare to read a memoir of an alcoholic, or food or drug addict, who has made no improvement. Written accounts rarely end with the author claiming that they found themselves in a worse place than they began. Yet, these 'health failures', for want of a better phrase, undoubtedly do exist and are part of everyday health experiences. We need to be acutely aware that, as ever, history prioritises the accounts of the victors.

The idea of archival silences also plays out within museums and heritage organisations. Collections might prioritise hegemonic perspectives, partly because their collections were gathered during a different historic time which cared little for cultural theft and largely catered for white, able-bodied audiences. Disease and illness are great equalisers, with the ability to transcend class, race and gender differences (except in very rare instances). Arguably, when developing and building health exhibits, it is, therefore, more important than ever for museum professionals to facilitate wide and inclusionary access. This can be done via careful consideration of exhibition content and messaging, but also by paying attention to physical museum access, exhibition design (signage and positioning) and pricing.

Some Limitations to Using Oral History

The way oral history relies upon listening, sympathy, cooperation and breaking down traditional hierarchies means that participating in oral history can benefit both the interviewer and the interviewee. Yet, certain challenges do exist and it is important to be cognisant of these when listening to oral histories retrospectively or when making oral histories either as the one telling their story or the one capturing it.

First, the taking of oral histories brings ethical challenges. These centre on the way oral history subjects might be perceived as being in a vulnerable position vis-á-vis the 'powerful' role of the interviewer. All interviews, however informal or self-consciously designed to be democratic and unthreatening, nevertheless play to some degree into a power dynamic where one person is actively collecting the information that they want and the other is supplying it. This means interviewees might sometimes adapt their narrative responses to suit what they feel their interviewer *wants to hear*. In a similar vein, family, professional or other contextual considerations might influence an interviewee's ability to talk frankly or honestly. In situations where participants have had a health experience, the revelation of which might impact other people, oral history needs

to be deployed carefully. Subjects may be worried about disclos-
ing their health stories frankly, especially if these touch upon their
'sexuality, drug use, lifestyle, illicit activities or experiences of violence' (Rickard, 1998, p. 41).[2]

Problems with Partnerships

Although Chapter 3 described many examples of the ways historians have successfully worked with policymakers, the integration
of history into the policy-making arena is not without practical
problems. As Sheard (2008) pointed out:

> They [historians] have usually been involved on a 'need to
> know' basis .... The use of experts in policy formation is
> a long-established principle – but too often history is not
> recognised as expert knowledge, or else it is provided by
> existing health professional staff who feel that their ama-
> teur interest gives them the confidence and authority to
> take this role on themselves. (p. 740)[3]

Virginia Berridge has highlighted similar challenges. She has
critiqued policymakers and politicians for using history in a 'cava-
lier' manner – describing them as too keen to quote statistics or
revert to simplistic readings of the past which serve their current
agendas (Berridge, 2016, p. 118).[4] Although health policymakers
do invoke historical precedents to support their policy initiatives,
the effectiveness of these invocations has been inconsistent. In part,
this is because policymakers and historians do not speak quite the
same language, embody the same objectives or work on the same
time scales. Although Berridge noted that most people working in
policy-related positions were favourably disposed, in theory, to historians and their work, her analysis concluded that actual engagement ultimately remained quite superficial, tending especially to
avoid thinking about the role of historical interpretation and how
and why one narrative becomes prioritised above another. History
used by policymakers is therefore often deployed in an essential-
ist, self-serving way. More often than not, historians are not even
involved at all.

Partnerships in the realm of public history can also bring challenges. To maximise the impact of a historical message, it is important for exhibition curators, film directors and professional historians to work in tandem with those who are going to disseminate their history. A public health message, for example, is much more effective if the partners have some knowledge about the public health issues raised and they actively help to facilitate access to networks that can raise the profile of the organisation by showing the exhibition or disseminating the public history resource (film, documentary and workshop). One of the challenges inherent in partnerships is reconciling divergent views as to what will work, or not. In the case of museums, there might be tensions where the museum professionals do not want to be beholden to external authorities guiding how an exhibition or outreach programme should be rolled out. Or discord might emerge where a publisher has slightly different views of the author. Similarly, a media production team's ideas might differ from the vision of a director or participant. It is impossible to predict accurately what the points of conflict might be in any given scenario, but it is not hard to envisage a situation where the body delivering the public health history exhibition or film is more concerned with creating a narrative and visual feast whereas the health-related professionals may be more invested in technical accuracy and tangibly tracking health behavioural changes.

ORAL HISTORY AS A FIRST STEP FOR ENGAGEMENT

If this book has shown anything, I would hope it has shown how deeply history permeates everyone's sense of self, not only influencing how many of us choose to spend our leisure time but also running powerfully through the bigger structures of society in which we are embedded and the professional lives many of us lead. It is not hard to engage with history for health. People can visit a museum or heritage site, read a history book, watch a historical documentary or flick through an old family album. Visiting an archive is also usually pretty straightforward and archivists are without exception some of the most helpful and enthusiastic professionals

I have ever met. In the next chapter (Chapter 6), I list a range of resources that I hope people will find useful to get started in thinking about the relationship between history, health and wellbeing. Before moving on to that chapter, however, I pause briefly to reiterate the value of oral histories as a first step for engagement with 'history for health' and to highlight the rich opportunities available in oral history resources.

Many important and growing oral history archives relating to health and wellbeing are available in the UK. A large corpus is located at the British Library, London, which includes digitised collections by *National Life Stories*, an independent charitable trust (founded in 1987) whose specific remit is to gather and preserve oral histories. While some of the British Library collections record the experiences of medical professionals (from researchers to clinicians, to nurses, to pharmacists, to counsellors and psychotherapists), others present the experiences of those with disabilities or those who have lived with physical and/or mental ill-health, including those who lived during the 1980s AIDs epidemic or in its aftermath, and life stories of those living with diabetes, multiple sclerosis and mental health diagnoses.[5] Other regional UK collections also provide important resources. Here, I am particularly thinking of the oral history centre at the University of Essex, which holds particularly strong collections on LGBTQ+ histories, disability, war and Black history.[6]

In the USA, a number of important collections deserve mention. The full list is too large to mention but includes oral histories housed in the United States Food and Drug Administration collection and the practitioners of homeopathic medicine collection at the National Library of Medicine, Bethesda, Maryland. Large digitised oral history collections also exist at the Center for Oral History at the Science History Institute, headquartered in Philadelphia, Pennsylvania. The Becker Library in St Louis, Missouri, houses collections for the Washington University School of Medicine Oral History project, with interviews and transcripts dating back to 1959. The Baylor College of Medicine in Houston, Texas and the Regional Oral History Office at the University of California at Berkeley also hold large and important collections.

Online there is also an abundance of collections that can be accessed easily from the comfort of your home. Websites such as *Healthtalk* provide thousands of filmed experiences of what it is like to live with a particular health condition, from menopause to psychosis.[7] Similarly, *Inside Stories of Mental Health Care* provides many interviews pertaining to those who have had mental health conditions.[8]

The recorded testimony of victims of disaster, displacement and trauma are also available via online sites. The *September 11 Digital Archive* contains more than 40,000 first-hand stories.[9] Steven Spielberg's *Survivors of the Shoah* web archive (mentioned in Chapter 2) hosts interviews with nearly 55,000 Holocaust survivors.[10]

Oral history collections can be an ongoing thing, creating living archives that grow year by year. To this end, some charities see the value of collecting narratives, as evidenced by the 'tell us your story' offer on the Diabetes UK website, which encourages people to add their subjective narratives 'to help or encourage others'.[11] More recently started is the *NHS Voices of COVID-19* project led by Professor Stephanie Snow, University of Manchester, in partnership with the British Library and funded by the Arts and Humanities Research Council. This project aims to collect 900 oral testimonies of people's experiences during and since the COVID-19 pandemic.[12] This will become a vastly important archive of the future, providing insights into how we coped with the pandemic and its effects.

Finally, it is worth mentioning just a few of the very large number of academic books which centrally draw on oral historical evidence to substantiate their health histories. The field, once again, is too large to mention more than a handful, but this is an area where those interested in seeing how historians have interpreted oral evidence can reap fruitful rewards. Monographs (listed in the bibliography at the end of Chapter 6) range from books which analyse interviews with doctors and policymakers involved in early AIDS/HIV responses (Bayer & Oppenheimer, 2000; Berridge, 1996) to collections which present testimonies of those who live with HIV and AIDS (Richardson & Bolle, 2017). There are oral histories of NHS general practitioners (Bevan, 2000) and cardiologists and surgeons working in the field of heart disease (Weisse, 2002).

Oral testimony has also been collected to bring new life to nursing history (Mitchell & Rafferty, 2005; Russell, 1997; Zalumas, 1995). Oral histories of homosexuality have looked back to a time when gay sexual orientation was regarded as unhealthy and to be remedially treated (Smith, Bartlett, & King, 2004).

When reaching across time for health consolation and information, oral history provides one of the most helpful bridges between academic analysis and lived experience. It inspires connectivity, but perhaps even more importantly, it presents us with a portfolio of possibilities into which we can dive, if not for definitive answers, then for succour. I urge readers to sample from the large range of oral testimonies available.

NOTES

1. Bønnelycke, J., Grabowski, D., Christensen, J. H., Bentsen, P., & Jespersen, A. P. (2021). Health, fun and ontonorms: Museums promoting health and physical activity. *Museum Management and Curatorship*, 36(3), 286–302. https://doi.org/10.1080/09647775.2020.1723132.

2. Rickard, W. (1998). Oral history – 'More dangerous than therapy'?: Interviewees' reflections on recording traumatic or taboo issues. *Oral History*, 26(2), 34–48. Retrieved from https://www.jstor.org/stable/40179520.

3. Sheard, S. (2008). History in health and health services: Exploring the possibilities. *Journal of Epidemiology & Community Health*, 62(8), 740–744. http://dx.doi.org/10.1136/jech.2007.063412.

4. Berridge, V. (2016). History and the future: Looking back to look forward? *International Journal of Drug Policy*, 37, 117–121. https://doi.org/10.1016/j.drugpo.2016.09.002.

5. British Library. (n.d.) Oral histories of medicine and health professionals. Retrieved from https://www.bl.uk/collection-guides/oral-histories-of-medicine-and-health-professionals; British Library. (n.d.) Oral histories of disability and personal and mental health. Retrieved from https://www.bl.uk/collection-guides/oral-histories-of-personal-and-mental-health-and-disability.

6. University of Essex, Library & Cultural Services. (n.d.). Oral history collections. Retrieved from https://library.essex.ac.uk/history/oralhistory.

7. healthtalk.org. (n.d.). Retrieved from https://healthtalk.org.

8. The Testimony archive. (n.d.). An oral history of mental health care. Retrieved from https://www.webarchive.org.uk/wayback/archive/2 0121113104505/http://insidestories.org/archive.

9. The September 11 Digital Archive. (n.d.). Retrieved from https://911digitalarchive.org.

10. USC Shoah Foundation. (n.d.). Retrieved from https://sfi.usc.edu.

11. Diabetes UK. (n.d.). Retrieved from https://www.diabetes.org.uk/ your-stories.

12. NHS Voices of COVID-19. (n.d.). Retrieved from https://www.nhs70. org.uk/covidvoices.

6

CONCLUSIONS, USEFUL LINKS AND FURTHER READING

The constitution of the World Health Organization declares that 'good health is a state of complete physical, social and mental wellbeing, and not merely the absence of disease or infirmity'.[1] With this definition in mind, good health is a state of wellbeing in which an individual realises their own abilities, can cope with the normal stresses of life, can work productively, is largely accepting of themselves and can make a contribution to their community. There are several ways people can work towards achieving this ideal mental health status. For many, seeing a doctor, psychiatrist, psychologist or other mental health professional offers important therapeutic avenues which range from talking therapies to psychopharmaceuticals. But roads to good health are broader than these clinical approaches. As social prescribing increasingly attests, participating in the arts or in community projects or pursuing an outdoor activity, are also important boosters of wellbeing.

The arts and humanities in general, and history specifically, can act to humanise some of the more institutionalised parts of medicine and caring. As concluded in a recent report on the importance of museums and galleries for health and wellbeing, taking a wellbeing allowance, even if just 30 minutes a day, 'can work wonders' in managing the stresses of modern life (Deuchar, 2019).[2] Similar research has not yet been systematically conducted on the health benefits of immersing oneself in family memories, or researching family genealogy, reading history books, or listening to oral history recordings, but these too offer a diversity of emotional benefits. Engaging with history can be affirming, sociable, distracting, calming, educative, liberating and healing.

It is notable that history has never really been singled out as a discipline of importance in relation to health. I truly think that this is because it is so embedded in all the things we do, to the point that we are often not conscious that we are encountering history. Every gallery we go to, each cityscape we admire, every book we read, every story we tell (or hear) involves history to some extent. Politicians, policymakers and polemicists draw on history all the time – even if they sometimes do so without precision. History can be a stimulus for change, as well as a prophetic warning of what might happen. Essentially, without even knowing it, people care about history, even if they did not enjoy it at school or do not identify themselves as historians. Delving into the past offers scaffolding to people's present. History can highlight the importance of locality and culture in every interaction. Past experiences alert us to possibilities that we may not have thought of. History can show us that change is possible or that things are better now.

Our health is bound up in history: in the history of technology and pharmacology, in histories of medical discoveries and developments, but also in histories of pain, suffering, trauma, survival, birth and demise. How we experience our own ill-health, or the illnesses of others, is irrevocably connected to attitudes and precedents of the past. History is particularly helpful to those with uncertain health conditions because it offers its readers and listeners a means of embracing the uncertainty and complexity of past decisions, actions and feelings. It teaches us to be questioning of some of the information we are given and to examine alternative ways of looking at things. To refer to words used by American historian, J Franklin Jameson, in his address to the trustees of the Carnegie Institute, Washington DC, in 1912: history 'will always make an invaluable foe of credulity, the steady propagator of that methodological doubt on which enlightenment so largely depends' (Jameson, 1912).[3] These interrogative skills promote a healthy scepticism and also show how mutable the past is, dependent on who is interpreting it, how they do so and why.

History interprets the human condition, of which health and caring are perhaps the most vital elements. History can deepen sympathies, extend imaginations and create therapeutic communities beyond the customary restrictions of geography and time.

NOTES

1. World Health Organization. Constitution. Retrieved from https://www.who.int/about/governance/constitution. Accessed on December 20, 2022.

2. Deuchar, S. (2019). *Calm and collected, museums and galleries: The UK's untapped wellbeing resource*. London: The Art Fund.

3. Jameson's quotation is taken from a paper he delivered in 1912 entitled 'The Future Uses of History', first published in 1913 in *The History Teacher's Magazine*, 4(2), and subsequently published in 1959 in *American Historical Review*, 65(1), 61–71 (see p. 62).

USEFUL LINKS AND REFERENCES

Due to restraints of space, UK collections have been prioritised (although others are mentioned).

KEY WEBSITES

Culture Health & Wellbeing Alliance. (n.d.). Retrieved from https://www.culturehealthandwellbeing.org.uk

History & Policy. (n.d.). Retrieved from https://www.historyandpolicy.org

Lapidus International (the Writing and Wellbeing Community). (n.d.). Retrieved from https://www.lapidus.org.uk

National Academy for Social Prescribing. (n.d.). Retrieved from https://socialprescribingacademy.org.uk

National Library of Medicine, Bethesda, Maryland, USA. (n.d.). Retrieved from https://www.nlm.nih.gov/hmd/collections/index.html

Society for the Social History of Medicine. (n.d.). Retrieved from https://
sshm.org/portfolio/the-society/

Wellcome Trust Library, London, UK. (n.d.). Retrieved from https://
wellcomecollection.org/collections

CITED ONLINE REPORTS AND POLICY-RELATED PAPERS

Crimmins, P. (2022, June 14). Why visiting a museum is good for your
health. *WITF News*. Retrieved from https://www.witf.org/2022/06/14/
why-visiting-a-museum-is-good-for-your-health/

Desmarais, S., Bedford, L., & Chatterjee, H. J. (2018). Museums as spaces
for wellbeing: A second report from the National Alliance for Museums
and Wellbeing. Retrieved from https://museumsandwellbeingalliance.
files.wordpress.com/2018/04/museums-as-spaces-for-wellbeing-a-second-
report.pdf

Fox, J., Coast, D., & Forward, J. (2022). *Covid rumours in historical
context – Two policymaking paradigms*. History & Policy. Retrieved
from https://www.historyandpolicy.org/policy-papers/papers/
covid-rumours-in-historical-context-two-policymaking-paradigms

Gorsky, M. (2006). *Hospital governance and community involvement in
Britain: Evidence from before the National Health Service*. History &
Policy. Retrieved from https://www.historyandpolicy.org/policy-papers/
papers/hospital-governance-and-community-involvement-in-britain-
evidence-from-befo

Haggett, A. (2016). *Men, mental illness and suicide: The current
scene in historical context*. History & Policy. Retrieved from https://
www.historyandpolicy.org/policy-papers/papers/men-mental-illness-
and-suicide-the-current-scene-in-historical-context

Hearne, S. (2021). *Criminalising disease transmission: Lessons from
Soviet approaches to sexual health*. History & Policy. Retrieved from
https://www.historyandpolicy.org/policy-papers/papers/criminalising-
disease-transmission-lessons-from-soviet-approaches-to-sexual-health

Irving, H., Cresswell, R., Doyle, B., Ewen, S., Roodhouse, M., Tomlinson,
C., & Wiggam, M. (2020). *The real lessons of the Blitz for Covid-19*.

History & Policy. Retrieved from https://www.historyandpolicy.org/policy-papers/papers/the-real-lessons-of-the-blitz-for-covid-19

McGuire, C. (2020). *How technology has been used to deny benefits to the disabled*. History & Policy. Retrieved from https://www.historyandpolicy.org/policy-papers/papers/how-technology-has-been-used-to-deny-benefits-to-the-disabled

PolicyBristol. (2018). *More than a medical symptom: The need for holistic care of breathlessness*. Policy Report, 43. PolicyBristol. Retrieved from https://www.bristol.ac.uk/policybristol/policy-briefings/life-of-breath/

Small, H. (2020). *Florence Nightingale's Public Health Act, Covid-19 and the empowerment of local government*. History & Policy. Retrieved from https://www.historyandpolicy.org/policy-papers/papers/florence-nightingales-public-health-act-covid-19-and-the-empowerment-of-local-government

PERSONAL BLOGS

Tammy Tour Guide. (2014, May 19). The museum diet – How to lose weight on holiday. Retrieved from https://tammytourguide.wordpress.com/2014/05/19/the-museum-diet-and-how-to-lose-weight-on-holiday/

FAMILY HISTORY RESOURCES

Ancestry.com (UK site). (n.d.). Retrieved from www.ancestry.co.uk

Barnardo's Making Connections. (n.d.). Retrieved from https://www.barnardos.org.uk/former-barnardos-children

British Home Children Registry. (n.d.). Retrieved from http://britishhomechildrenregistry.com

Children's Home Residence Lists (UK). (n.d.). Retrieved from www.childrenshomes.org.uk

Civil Registrations in England and Wales. (n.d.). Retrieved from https://www.freebmd.org.uk/

Convict Transportation Records (Australia). (n.d.). Retrieved from www.ancestry.com.au

Donor and Genetic Children Register. (n.d.). Retrieved from https://www.
liverpoolwomens.nhs.uk/our-services/donor-conceived-register-dcr/

General Register Office. (n.d.). Retrieved from www.gro.gov.uk

Hospital Records Database (via National Archives). (n.d.). Retrieved from
https://discovery.nationalarchives.gov.uk

Mental Health Institutions Records. (n.d.). Retrieved from https://
museumofthemind.org.uk/collections/archives

National Records of Scotland. (n.d.). Retrieved from www.
scotlandspeople.gov.uk

POLICY REPORTS

Deuchar, S. (2019). *Calm and collected, museums and galleries: The UK's
untapped wellbeing resource.* The Art Fund.

Johnston, R., & McIvor, A. (2001). *Oral histories of the asbestos tragedy
in Scotland.* Report for International Ban Asbestos Secretariat. Retrieved
from http://ibasecretariat.org/eas_rj_am_scotland.php

Lampard, K., & Marsden, E. (2015). *Themes and lessons learnt from
NHS investigations into matters relating to Jimmy Savile.* Independent
report for the Secretary of State for Health. Retrieved from https://
assets.publishing.service.gov.uk/government/uploads/system/uploads/
attachment_data/file/407209/KL_lessons_learned_report_FINAL.pdf

NHS Long Term Plan. (2019). Retrieved from https://www.longtermplan.
nhs.uk

NHS Self-help Guide to Mental Wellbeing. (2022). Retrieved from
https://www.nhs.uk/mental-health/self-help/guides-tools-and-activities/
five-steps-to-mental-wellbeing/

MUSEUMS AND EXHIBITIONS, PROJECTS AND ARCHIVES

Breaking Ground Heritage. (n.d.). Retrieved from https://
breakinggroundheritage.org.uk

Creative Carers Programme, Birmingham Museums Trust. (n.d.).
Retrieved from https://forwardcarers.org.uk/creative-carers-
programme/

The Gurkha Connection Project, Hampshire Cultural Trust. (n.d.).
Retrieved from https://www.hampshireculture.org.uk/social-impact/
gurkha-connection

House of Memories, Dementia Awareness Programme, Liverpool
Museums. (n.d.). Retrieved from https://www.liverpoolmuseums.org.uk/
house-of-memories/about

Meet Me: The MoMA Alzheimer's Project: Making Art Accessible to
People with Dementia. (n.d.). Retrieved from https://www.moma.org/visit/
accessibility/meetme/index.html

Ministry of Defence, Operation Nightingale. (n.d.). Retrieved from
https://www.gov.uk/guidance/operation-nightingale

The Life of Breath. (n.d.). Retrieved from www.lifeofbreath.org

The Museum as a Gym: Fitness trail at the Kunsthaus Graz, Austria.
(n.d.). Retrieved from https://www.museum-joanneum.at/en/kunsthaus-
graz/exhibitions/art-projects/temporary-projects/events/event/5130/
the-museum-as-a-gym-3

Science Museum London. (n.d.). Retrieved from https://www.
sciencemuseum.org.uk

US American Veterans Archaeology programme. (n.d.). Retrieved from
https://americanveteransarchaeology.org/

Waterloo Uncovered. (n.d.). Retrieved from https://waterloouncovered.
com/about/

Wessex Archaeology, Operation Nightingale. (n.d.). Retrieved from
https://www.wessexarch.co.uk/our-work/operation-nightingale

ORAL HISTORY COLLECTIONS (ONLINE)

British Library. (n.d.). Oral histories of disability and personal and
mental health. Retrieved from https://www.bl.uk/collection-guides/
oral-histories-of-personal-and-mental-health-and-disability

British Library. (n.d.). Oral histories of medicine and health professionals. Retrieved from https://www.bl.uk/collection-guides/oral-histories-of-medicine-and-health-professionals

Diabetes UK. (n.d.). Your stories. Retrieved from https://www.diabetes.org.uk/your-stories

Glenside Hospital Museum. (n.d.). Bristol oral history collections. Retrieved from https://www.glensidemuseum.org.uk

Health Talk. (n.d.). Real people, real life experiences. Retrieved from https://healthtalk.org

Johnston, R., & McIvor, A. (2001). *Oral histories of the asbestos tragedy in Scotland*. Report for International Ban Asbestos Secretariat. Retrieved from http://ibasecretariat.org/eas_rj_am_scotland.php

NHS Voices of Covid-19. (n.d.). Retrieved from https://www.nhs70.org.uk/covidvoices

Royal College of Nurses Archive, Edinburgh. (n.d.). Oral history collection. Retrieved from https://www.rcn.org.uk/library-exhibitions/special-collections-oral-history

Royal College of Physicians, London. (n.d.). Oral history collection. Retrieved from https://history.rcplondon.ac.uk/collections/oral-history

The September 11 Digital Archive. Retrieved from https://911digitalarchive.org

The Shoah Foundation (oral testimony of holocaust survivors). (n.d.). Retrieved from https://sfi.usc.edu

The Testimony Archive: Inside Stories of Mental Health. (n.d.). Archived website. Retrieved from https://www.webarchive.org.uk/wayback/archive/20121113104505/http://insidestories.org/archive

University of Essex, Library and Cultural Services. (n.d.). Oral history collection. Retrieved from https://library.essex.ac.uk/history/oralhistory

Wellcome Trust, London. (n.d.). Oral history collection. Retrieved from https://wellcomecollection.org/collections, including the Witnesses to Twentieth Century Medicine Seminars: https://wellcomecollection.org/works/fsyrn6bu

ORAL HISTORIES (IN BOOKS AND JOURNALS)

Bayer, R., & Oppenheimer, G. M. (2002). *AIDS doctors: Voices from the epidemic: An oral history*. Oxford: Oxford University Press.

Berridge, V. (1996). *AIDS in the UK: The making of a policy, 1981–1994*. Oxford: Oxford University Press.

Bevan, M. (2000). Family and vocation: Career choice and the life histories of general practitioners. In J. Bornat, R. Perks, P. Thompson, & J. Walmsley (Eds.), *Oral history, health and welfare* (pp. 21–46). London: Psychology Press.

Mitchell, D., & Rafferty, A. M. (2005). I don't think they ever really wanted to know anything about us: Oral history interviews with learning disability nurses. *Oral History, 33*(1), 77–87. Retrieved from https://e-space.mmu.ac.uk/id/eprint/84221

Richardson, A., & Bolle, D. (2017). *Wise before their time: People with AIDS and HIV talk about their lives*. Independently published.

Rivers, T. M. (1967). *Tom Rivers: Reflections on a life in medicine and science: An oral history memoir*. Cambridge, MA: The MIT Press.

Russell, D. (1997). An oral history project in mental health nursing. *Journal of Advanced Nursing, 26*(3), 489–495. https://doi.org/10.1046/j.1365-2648.1997.t01-7-00999.x

Smith, G., Bartlett, A., & King, M. (2004). Treatments of homosexuality in Britain since the 1950s—An oral history: The experience of patients. *British Medical Journal, 328*(7437), 42. https://doi.org/10.1136%2Fbmj.37984.442419.EE

Weisse, A. B. (2002). *Heart to heart: The twentieth century battle against cardiac disease: An oral history*. New Brunswick: Rutgers University Press.

Zalumas, J. (1995). *Caring in crisis: An oral history of critical care nursing*. Philadelphia: University of Pennsylvania Press.

ACADEMIC HEALTH HISTORIES

Anderson, D. (2005). *Histories of the hanged: The dirty war in Kenya and the end of empire*. New York, NY: WW Norton.

Berridge, V. (2007). *Marketing health: Smoking and the discourse of public health in Britain, 1945–2000*. Oxford: Oxford University Press.

Bourke, J. (2014). *The story of pain: From prayer to painkillers*. Oxford: Oxford University Press.

Brandt, A. (2009). *Cigarette century: The rise, fall, and deadly persistence of the product that defined America*. New York, NY: Basic Books.

Braun, L., (2014). *Breathing race into the machine: The surprising career of the spirometer from plantation to genetics*. Minneapolis, MN: University of Minnesota Press.

Bryant, K. (2020). *Hysteria: A memoir of illness, strength and women's stories throughout history*. Sydney: Newsouth Books.

Burch, S., & Rembis, M. (Eds.). (2014). *Disability histories*. Champaign: University of Illinois Press.

Bynum, H. (2015). *Spitting blood: The history of tuberculosis*. Oxford: Oxford University Press.

Cleghorn, E., (2021). *Unwell women: A journey through medicine and myth in a man-made world*. London: Weidenfeld & Nicolson.

Courtwright, D. (2019). *The age of addiction: How bad habits became big business*. Cambridge, MA: Harvard University Press.

Downs, J. (2021). *Maladies of empire: How colonialism, slavery, and war transformed medicine*. Cambridge, MA: Harvard University Press.

Durbach, N. (2010). *Spectacle of deformity: Freak shows and modern British culture*. Oakland, CA: University of California Press.

Elkins, C. (2005). *Imperial reckoning: The untold story of Britain's gulag in Kenya*. New York, NY: Henry Holt & Co.

Elkins, C. (2014). *Britain's gulag: The brutal end of empire in Kenya*. Oxford: The Bodley Head.

Heyam, K. (2022). *Before we were trans: A new history of gender*. New York, NY: Basic Books.

Hutchinson, I., Atherton, M., & Virdi, J. (2020). *Disability and the Victorians: Attitudes, interventions, legacies*. Manchester: Manchester University Press.

Langer, L. (1993). *Holocaust testimonies: The ruins of memory*. New Haven, CT: Yale University Press.

Lougheed, K. (2017). *Catching breath: The making and unmaking of tuberculosis*. London: Bloomsbury Sigma.

McGuire, C. (2019a). 'X-rays don't tell lies': The Medical Research Council and the measurement of respiratory disability, 1936–1945. *British Journal for the History of Science*, 52(3), 447–465. https://doi.org/10.1017/S0007087419000232

McGuire, C., (2019b). Dust to dust. *The Lancet Respiratory Medicine*, 7(5), 383–384. https://doi.org/10.1016/S2213-2600(19)30116-X

McGuire, C. (2020). *Measuring difference, numbering normal: Setting the standards for disability in the interwar period*. Manchester: Manchester University Press.

McGuire, C., Macnaughton, J., & Carel, H., (2020). The color of breath. *Literature and Medicine*, 38(2), 233–238. http://doi.org/10.1353/lm.2020.0015

McKay, R. (2017). *Patient zero and the making of the AIDS epidemic*. Chicago, IL: University of Chicago Press.

Metzl, J. M. (2010). *The protest psychosis: How schizophrenia became a black disease*. Boston, MA: Beacon Press.

Moscucci, O. (2016). *Gender and cancer in England, 1860–1948*. London: Palgrave Macmillan.

Myerhoff, B. G. (1994, first published 1978). *Number our days: Culture and community among elderly Jews in an American ghetto*. New York, NY: Plume.

Myers, D. N. (2018). *The stakes of history: On the use and abuse of Jewish history for life*. New Haven, CT: Yale University Press.

O'Neill, D., & Greenwood, A. (2022, August 11). "Bringing you the best": John Player & Sons, cricket and the politics of tobacco sport sponsorship in Britain, 1969–1986. *European Journal for the History of Medicine and Health*, advance online publication. https://doi.org/10.1163/26667711-bja10022

Ophir, O. (2022). *Schizophrenia: An unfinished history*. Polity Cambridge: Books.

Proctor, R. (2011). *Golden holocaust: Origins of the cigarette catastrophe and the case for abolition.* Oakland, CA: University of California Press.

Reverby, S. M. (2009). *Examining Tuskegee: The infamous syphilis study and its legacy.* Chapel Hill, NC: University of North Carolina Press.

Scull, A. (2022). *Desperate remedies: Psychiatry and the mysteries of mental illness.* London: Allen Lane.

Sheard, S., & Donaldson, L. (2018, first published 2006). *The nation's doctor: The role of the Chief Medical Officer 1855–1998.* Boca Raton, FL: CRC Press.

Snorton, C. R. (2017). *Black on both sides: A racial history of trans identity.* Minneapolis, MN: University of Minnesota Press.

Sontag, S. (1978). *Illness as metaphor.* New York, NY: Farrar, Straus & Giroux.

Strings, S. (2019). *Fearing the black body: The racial origins of fat phobia.* New York, NY: New York University Press.

Stryker, S. (2017). *Transgender history: The roots of today's revolution.* New York, NY: Hachette.

Timmermann, C., & E. Toon (2012). *Cancer patients, cancer pathways: Historical and sociological perspectives.* London: Palgrave Macmillan.

Washington, H. A. (2006). *Medical apartheid: The dark history of medical experimentation on Black Americans from colonial times to the present.* New York, NY: Doubleday Books.

Weston, J., & Elizabeth H. J. (2022). *Histories of HIV/AIDS in Western Europe: New and regional perspectives.* Manchester: Manchester University Press.

Zeldin, T. (1995). *An intimate history of humanity.* New York, NY: Harper Collins.

POPULAR AND PERSONAL HEALTH HISTORIES AND PERSONAL MEMOIRS

Adams, T. (1998). *Addicted.* London: Collins Willow.

Allen, C. (1978). *I'm Black and I'm sober: The timeless story of a woman's journey back to sanity*. Minnesota, MN: Hazelden.

Atkins, E. (1994). *One door closes another opens: A personal experience of polio*. London: Waltham Forest Oral History Workshop.

Barry, J. (2005). *The great influenza: The story of the deadliest pandemic in history*. New York, NY: Penguin Books.

Brown, A. (2019). *The prison doctor: My time inside Britain's most notorious jails*. London: HarperCollins.

Burroughs, W. (writing as William Lee) (1953). *Junkie: Confessions of an unredeemed drug addict*. New York, NY: Ace Books.

Chan, A., & Ridley, M. (2021). *Viral: The search for the origin of Covid-19*. London: HarperCollins.

Crowley, A. (1922). *Diary of a Drug Fiend*. London: Collins.

De Quincey, T. (1823). *Confessions of an English Opium-Eater*. London: Taylor and Hessey.

De Rossi, P. (2010). *Unbearable lightness: A story of loss and gain*. New York, NY: Simon and Schuster.

Fitzharris, L. (2018). *The butchering art: Joseph Lister's quest to transform the grisly world of Victorian medicine*. London: Penguin Books.

Fitzharris, L. (2022). *The facemaker: A visionary surgeon's battle to mend the disfigured soldiers of World War I*. New York, NY: Farrar, Straus and Giroux.

Gray, C. (2017). *The unexpected joy of being sober*. London: Aster.

Hornbacher, M. (1998). *Wasted: A memoir of anorexia and bulimia*. London: Flamingo.

Hyung-Oak Lee, C. (2017). *Tell me everything you don't remember: The stroke that changed my life*. New York, NY: HarperCollins.

Johnson, S. (2007). *The ghost map: The story of London's most terrifying epidemic and how it changed science, cities and the modern world*. New York, NY: Riverhead Books.

Kay, A. (2017). *This is going to hurt: Secret diaries of a junior doctor*. London: Picador.

Kelly, J. (2006). *The great mortality: An intimate history of the black death, the most devastating plague of all time.* New York, NY: Harper Perennial.

Khakpour, P. (2018). *Sick.* Edinburgh: Canongate Books.

London, J. (1913). *John Barleycorn: Alcoholic memoirs.* London: Mills & Boon.

Lorde, A. (1997). *The cancer journals.* San Francisco, CA: Aunt Lute Books.

Meozzi, M. (2014). *Haldol and hyacinths: A bipolar life.* New York, NY: Avery.

Mukherjee, S. (2011). *The emperor of all maladies: A biography of cancer.* London: Fourth Estate.

Petersen, A. (2018). *On the edge: A journey through anxiety.* New York, NY: Broadway Books.

Pickert, K. (2019). *Radical: The science, culture and history of breast cancer in America.* Boston, MA: Little, Brown Spark.

Rice-Oxley, M. (2012). *Underneath the lemon tree: A memoir of depression and recovery.* Boston, MA: Little, Brown Spark.

Sanghera, S. (2009). *The boy with a topknot: A memoir of love, secrets and lies in Wolverhampton.* London: Penguin Books.

Sheff, D. (2008). *Beautiful Boy: A father's journey through his son's addiction.* Boston, MA: Houghton Mifflin.

Spinney, L. (2017). *Pale rider: The Spanish flu of 1918 and how it changed the world.* Public Affairs. London: Vintage.

METHODOLOGY, CRITICISM AND FINDINGS

Abrams, L. (2016). *Oral history theory.* London: Taylor and Francis.

Ackerman, A. (2016). Museums and health: A case study of research and practice at the Children's Museum of Manhattan. *Journal of Museum Education, 41*(2), 82–90. https://doi.org/10.1080/10598650. 2016.1169727

Baron, K. C., & Levstik, L. S. (2004). *Teaching history for the common good*. London: Routledge.

Baruch, J. M. (2017). Doctors as makers. *Academic Medicine, 92*(1), 40–44. https://doi.org/10.1097/acm.0000000000001312

Bashforth, M. (2012). Absent fathers, present histories. In P. Ashton & H. Kean (Eds.), *Public history and heritage today: People and their pasts* (pp. 203–222). London: Palgrave Macmillan.

Baum, W. (1981). Therapeutic value of oral history. *The International Journal of Aging and Human Development, 12*(1), 49–53. https://doi.org/10.2190/bype-ee50-j1tp-hv2v

Beauchet, O., Cooper-Brown, L., Hayashi, Y., Galery, K., Vilcocq, C., & Bastien, T. (2020). Effects of "Thursdays at the Museum" at the Montreal Museum of Fine Arts on the mental and physical health of older community dwellers: The art-health randomized clinical trial protocol. *Trials, 21*(1), 1–12. https://doi.org/10.1186/s13063-020-04625-3

Belgrave, B. (2012). Something borrowed, something new: History and the Waitangi Tribunal. In P. Ashton & H. Kean (Eds.), *Public history and heritage today: People and their pasts* (pp. 311–322). London: Palgrave Macmillan.

Berridge, V. (2003). Public or policy understanding of history. *Social History of Medicine, 16*(3), 511–523. https://doi.org/10.1093/shm/16.3.511

Berridge, V. (2008). History matters? History's role in health policy making. *Medical History, 52*(3), 311–326. https://doi.org/10.1017/S0025727300000168

Berridge, V. (2010). 'Hidden from history'?: Oral history and the history of health policy. *Oral History, 38*(1), 91–100. https://www.jstor.org/stable/40650319

Berridge, V. (2016). History and the future: Looking back to look forward? *International Journal of Drug Policy, 37*, 117–121. https://doi.org/10.1016/j.drugpo.2016.09.002

Bhakta, N. R., Kaminsky, D. A., Bime, C., Thakur, N., Hall, G., McCormack, M., & Stanojevic, S. (2022). Addressing race in pulmonary function testing by aligning intent and evidence with practice and perception. *Chest*, *161*(1), 288–297. https://doi.org/10.1016/j. chest.2021.08.053

Bønnelycke, J., Grabowski, D., Christensen, J. H., Bentsen, P., & Jespersen, A. P. (2021). Health, fun and ontonorms: Museums promoting health and physical activity. *Museum Management and Curatorship*, *36*(3), 286–302. https://doi.org/10.1080/09647775.2020.1723132

Bornat, J. (Ed.). (1994). *Reminiscence reviewed: Evaluations, achievements, perspectives*. Maidenhead: Open University Press.

Bornat, J. (2002). Oral history as a social movement: Reminiscence and older people. In R. Perks & A. Thompson (Eds.), *The oral history reader* (pp. 203–219). London: Routledge.

Bornat, J., Perks, R., Thompson, P., & Walmsley, J. (Eds.). (2000). *Oral history, health and welfare*. London: Psychology Press.

Brandt, A. M. (2004). From analysis to advocacy: Crossing boundaries as a historian of health policy. In F. Huisman & J. H. Warner (Eds.), *Locating medical history* (pp. 460–484). Baltimore, MD: Johns Hopkins University Press.

Bullock, A. (1994). Has History ceased to be relevant? *The Historian*, *43*(104), 16–19.

Burnell, K. J., Coleman, P. G., & Hunt, N. (2010). Coping with traumatic memories: Second World War veterans' experiences of social support in relation to the narrative coherence of war memories. *Ageing & Society*, *30*(1), 57–78. https://doi.org/10.1017/S0144686X0999016X

Butterfield, H. (1931). *The Whig interpretation of history*. London: G Bell & Sons.

Camic, P. M., & Chatterjee, H. J. (2013). Museums and art galleries as partners for public health interventions. *Perspectives in Public Health*, *133*(1), 66–71. https://doi.org/10.1177/1757913912468523

Camic, P. M., Hulbert, S., & Kimmel, J. (2019). Museum object handling: A health-promoting community-based activity for dementia care. *Journal of Health Psychology*, *24*(6), 787–798. https://doi. org/10.1177/1359105316685899

Cave, M., & Sloan, S. M. (Eds.). (2014). *Listening on the edge: Oral history in the aftermath of crisis.* Oxford: Oxford University Press.

Chatterjee, H. J., Camic, P. M., Lockyer, B., & Thomson, L. J. M. (2018). Non-clinical community interventions: A systematised review of social prescribing schemes. *Arts & Health, 10*(2), 97–123. https://doi.org/10.10 80/17533015.2017.1334002

Chatterjee, H. J., Clini, C., Butler, B., Al-Nammari, F., Al-Asir, R., & Katona, C. (2020). Exploring the psychosocial impact of cultural interventions with displaced people. In E. Fiddian-Qasmiyeh (Ed.), *Refuge in a moving world: Tracing refugee and migrant journeys across disciplines* (pp. 323–345). London: UCL Press.

Chatterjee, H. J., & Noble, G. (2009). Object therapy: A student-selected component exploring the potential of museum object handling as an enrichment activity for patients in hospital. *Global Journal of Health Sciences, 1*(2), 42–49. http://dx.doi.org/10.5539/gjhs.v1n2p42

Chatterjee, H., & Noble, G. (2013). *Museums, health and well-being.* Farnham: Ashgate.

Chatterjee, H., Vreeland, S., & Noble, G. (2009). Museopathy: Exploring the healing potential of handling museum objects. *Museum and Society, 7*(3), 164–177. Retrieved from http://www.le.ac.uk/ms/m&s/Issue%2021/ chattergee-vreeland-noble.pdf

Chaudhury, H. (1999). Self and reminiscence of place: A conceptual study. *Journal of Aging and Identity, 4*(4), 231–253. https://doi.org/10.1023/ A:1022835109862

Clow, A., & Fredhoi, C. (2006). Normalisation of salivary cortisol levels and self-report stress by a brief lunchtime visit to an art gallery by London City workers. *Journal of Holistic Healthcare, 3*(2), 29–32. Retrieved from https://westminsterresearch.westminster.ac.uk/download/ e2f2c5a83af1a5bda4ba86cd1a0d0fc06038ba9c54491da6bbe893801773 94b7/196888/Clow_%26_fredhoi_2006_final.pdf

Cox, P. (2013). The future uses of history. *History Workshop Journal, 75*(1), 125–145. https://doi.org/10.1093/hwj/dbs007

Crawford, P., Brown, B., Baker, C., Tischler, V., & Adams, B. (2015). *Health humanities.* London: Palgrave Macmillan.

Crow, W., & Bowles, D. (2018). Empathy and analogy in museum education. *Journal of Museum Education, 43*(4), 342–348. https://doi.org/ 10.1080/10598650.2018.1529904

Davis, P., & F. Magee. (2020). *Arts for health: Reading.* Bingley: Emerald Publishing.

DeNil, B., & Janssens, P. (2020). Preserved heritage: Stories and objects for mental health patients. In T. Kador & H. Chatterjee (Eds.), *Object-based learning and well-being* (pp. 183–196). London: Routledge.

Dobat, A. S., & Dobat, A. S., (2020). Arkæologi som terapi: Metaldetektor hobbyen og mental sundhed i Danmark. *Arkæologisk Forum, 43*, 11–24. Retrieved from http://www.archaeology.dk/17011/ Nr.%2043%20-%202020

Dobat, A. S., Dobat, A. S., & Schmidt, S. (2022). Archaeology as "self-therapy": Case studies of metal detecting communities in Britain and Denmark. In P. Everill & K. Burnell (Eds.), *Archaeology, heritage, and wellbeing* (pp. 145–161). London: Routledge.

Dobat, A. S., Wood, S. O., Jensen, B. S., Schmidt, S., & Dobat, A. S., (2020). "I now look forward to the future, by finding things from our past ... " Exploring the potential of metal detector archaeology as a source of well-being and happiness for British Armed Forces veterans with mental health impairments. *International Journal of Heritage Studies, 26*(4), 370–386. https://doi.org/10.1080/13527258.2019.1639069

Dodd, J., & Jones, C. (2014). *Mind, body, spirit: How museums impact health and wellbeing.* Leicester: Research Centre for Museums and Galleries.

Dudley, S. H. (2013). Museum materialities: Objects, sense and feeling. In S. H. Dudley (Ed.), *Museum materialities: Objects, engagements, interpretations* (pp. 21–38). London: Routledge.

Durant, W., & Durant, A. (1968). *The lessons of history.* New York, NY: Simon & Schuster.

Dyer, C. (2019). NHS pays £1.1m compensation to Jimmy Savile's victims. *British Medical Journal, 364.* https://doi.org/10.1136/bmj.l232

Edeiken, L. R. (1992). Children's museums: The serious business of wonder, play, and learning. *Curator: The Museum Journal, 35*(1), 21–27. https://doi.org/10.1111/j.2151-6952.1992.tb00731.x

Endacott, J., & Brooks, S. (2018). Historical empathy perspectives and responding to the past. In S. Alan (Ed.), *The Wiley international handbook of history teaching and learning* (pp. 203–225). Hoboken, NJ: Wiley.

Fancourt, D., & Steptoe, S. (2018). Physical and psychosocial factors in the prevention of chronic pain in older age. *The Journal of Pain, 19*(12), 1385–1391. https://doi.org/10.1016/j.jpain.2018.06.001

Foster, H. (2020). At the intersection of memory, history and story: An exploration of the nostalgic feelings that arose when listening to oral history archives as an inspiration for novel-writing. *LIRIC Journal, 1*(1), 86–107. https://www.researchgate.net/publication/355679224_At_the_ Intersection_of_Memory_History_and_Story_An_Exploration_of_the_ Nostalgic_Feeling_which_Arose_when_Listening_to_Oral_History_ Archives_as_an_Inspiration_for_Novel-Writing

Froggett, L., Farrier, A., & Poursanidou, K. (2011). *Who cares? Museums, health and wellbeing research Project: A study of the Renaissance Northwest Programme.* Preston: University of Central Lancashire.

Graham, J., Benson, L. M., Swanson, J., Potyk, D., Daratha, K., & Roberts, K. (2016). Medical humanities coursework is associated with greater measured empathy in medical students. *The American Journal of Medicine, 129*(12), 1334–1337. https://doi.org/10.1016/j. amjmed.2016.08.005

Green, A. (2015). History as expertise and the influence of political culture on advice for policy since Fulton. *Contemporary British History, 29*(1), 27–50. https://doi.org/10.1080/13619462.2014.953485

Green, A. (2016). *History, policy, and public purpose: Historians and historical thinking in government.* London: Palgrave Macmillan.

Green, S. H., Bayer, R., & Fairchild, A. L. (2016). Evidence, policy, and e-cigarettes—Will England reframe the debate? *New England Journal of Medicine, 374*(14), 1301–1303. https://doi.org/10.1056/nejmc1606395

Hamlin, C., & Sheard, S. (1998). Revolutions in public health: 1948, and 1998? *British Medical Journal*, *317*, 587–591. https://doi.org/10.1136%2 Fbmj.317.7158.587

Harvey, M. R., Mischler, E. G., Koenen, K., & Harney P. A. (2000). In the aftermath of sexual abuse: Making and remaking meaning in narratives of trauma and recovery. *Narrative Inquiry*, *10*(2), 291–311. https:// psycnet.apa.org/doi/10.1075/ni.10.2.02har

Henke, S. (2000). *Shattered subjects: Trauma and testimony in women's life-writing*. London: Palgrave Macmillan.

Hojat, M., Erdmann, J. B., & Gonnella, J. S. (2013). Personality assessments and outcomes in medical education and the practice of medicine: AMEE Guide No. 79. *Medical Teacher*, *35*, e1267–e1301. https://doi.org/10.3109/0142159x.2013.785654

Horrigan, B., Lewis, S., Abrams, D. I., & Pechura, C. (2012). Integrative medicine in America—How integrative medicine is being practiced in clinical centers across the United States. *Global Advances in Health and Medicine*, *1*(3), 18–94. https://doi.org/10.7453%2Fgahmj.2012. 1.3.006

Hunt, N., & Robbins, I. (1998). Telling stories of the war: Ageing veterans coping with their memories through narrative. *Oral History*, *26*(2), 57–64. https://www.jstor.org/stable/40179522

Jameson, F. J. (1959). The Future Uses of History. *American Historical Review*, *65*(1), 61–71 (reprint of 1912 speech).

Jordanova, L. (2019, first published 2000). *History in practice*. London: Bloomsbury Publishing.

Kaminsky, M. (2014, first published 1984). *The uses of reminiscence: New ways of working with older adults*. London: Routledge.

Kampourelli, V. (2022). Historical empathy and medicine: Pathography and empathy in Sophocles' Philoctetes. *Medicine, Health Care and Philosophy*, *25*, 561–575. https://doi.org/10.1007/s11019-022-10087-y

Kean, H. (2012). London stories: personal lives and public histories. In P. Ashton & H. Kean (Eds.), *Public history and heritage today: People and their pasts* (pp. 173–192). London: Palgrave Macmillan.

Koebner, I., Chatterjee, H., Witt, C., Tancredi, D., Rawal, R., Weinberg, G., & Meyers, F. (2022). The transition from in-person to virtual museum programming for individuals living with chronic pain – A formative evaluation. *Journal of Clinical and Translational Science*, 6(1), E58. https://doi.org/10.1017%2Fcts.2022.392

Koretzky, M. O. (2018). Seeing the present through the past: History, empathy, and medical education. *Journal of the American Medical Association*, 320(20), 2079–2080. https://doi.org/10.1001/jama.2018.17253

Labisch, A. (1998). History of public health—History in public health: Looking back and looking forward. *Social History of Medicine*, 11(1), 1–13. https://doi.org/10.1093/shm/11.1.1

Labisch, A. (2004). Transcending the two cultures in biomedicine: The history of medicine and history in medicine. In F. Huisman & J. H. Warner (Eds.), *Locating medical history: The stories and their meanings* (pp. 410–431). Baltimore, MD: Johns Hopkins University Press.

Langellier, K., & Peterson, E. (2004). *Storytelling in daily life: Performing narrative*. Philadelphia: Temple University Press.

Larsson, H., Rämgård, M., & Bolmsjö, I. (2017). Older persons' existential loneliness, as interpreted by their significant others – An interview study. *BMC Geriatrics*, 17(1), 1–9. https://doi.org/10.1186/s12877-017-0533-1

MacMillan, M. (2009). *The uses and abuses of history*. London: Profile Books.

Maggi, L. (2000). Bearing witness for tobacco. *Journal of Public Health Policy*, 21(3), 296–302. https://doi.org/10.2307/3343328

Markowitz, G., & Rosner, D. (2013, first published 2002). *Deceit and denial: The deadly politics of industrial pollution* (Vol. 6). Oakland, CA: University of California Press.

Marreez, Y. M. A. H., Willems, L. N., & Wells, M. R. (2010). The role of medical museums in contemporary medical education. *Anatomical Sciences Education*, 3(5), 249–253. https://doi.org/10.1002/ase.168

Mastandrea, S., Maricchiolo,F., Carrus, G., Giovannelli, I., Giuliani, V., & Berardi, B. (2018). Visits to figurative art museums may lower blood pressure and stress. *Arts & Health*, *11*(2), 123–132. https://doi.org/10.1080/17533015.2018.1443953

McLeary, E., & Toon, E. (2012). "Here man learns about himself": Visual education and the rise and fall of the American Museum of Health. *American Journal of Public Health*, *102*(7), e27–e36. http://dx.doi.org/10.2105/AJPH.2011.300560

Mendoza, N. (2017). *The Mendoza review: An independent review of museums in England*. London: Department for Digital, Culture, Media & Sport.

Morse, N., & Chatterjee, H. (2018). Museums, health and wellbeing research: Co-developing a new observational method for people with dementia in hospital contexts. *Perspectives in Public Health*, *138*(3), 152–159. https://doi.org/10.1177/1757913917737588

Morse, N., Thomson, L. J., Elsden, E., Rogers, H., & Chatterjee, H. J. (2022). Exploring the potential of creative museum-led activities to support stroke in-patient rehabilitation and wellbeing: A pilot mixed-methods study. *Arts & Health*, *15*(2), 135-152. https://doi.org/10.1080/17533015.2022.2032224

Mughal, R., Thomson, L. J. M., Daykin, N., & Chatterjee, H. J. (2022). Rapid evidence review of community engagement and resources in the UK during the COVID-19 pandemic: How can community assets redress health inequities? *International Journal of Environmental Research and Public Health*, *19*(7), 4086. https://doi.org/10.3390%2Fijerph19074086

Newman, J. (2012). Harry Jacobs: The studio photographer and the visual archive. In P. Ashton & H. Kean (Eds.), *Public history and heritage today: People and their pasts* (pp. 260–279). London: Palgrave Macmillan.

Perdiguero, E., Bernabeu, J., Huertas, R., & Rodríguez-Ocaña, E. (2001). History of health, a valuable tool in public health. *Journal of Epidemiology & Community Health*, *55*(9), 667–673. https://doi.org/10.1136%2Fjech.55.9.667

Perrotta, K., & Bohan, C. H. (2020). Can't stop this feeling: Tracing the origins of historical empathy during the Cold War era, 1950–1980.

Educational Studies, 56(6), 599–618. https://doi.org/10.1080/00131946.
2020.1837832

Porter, R. (1985). The patient's view. *Theory and Society, 14*(2), 175–198.
https://doi.org/10.1007/BF00157532

Porter, R. (1986). History says no to the policeman's response to AIDS.
British Medical Journal, 293, 1589–1590. https://doi.org/10.1136%2Fb
mj.293.6562.1589

Proctor, R. (2004). Should medical historians be working for the
tobacco industry? *The Lancet, 363*, 1174–1175. https://doi.org/10.1016/
s0140-6736(04)15981-3

Proctor, R. N. (2012). The history of the discovery of the cigarette–lung
cancer link: Evidentiary traditions, corporate denial, global toll.
Tobacco Control, 21(2), 87–91. https://doi.org/10.1136/tobaccocontrol-
2011-050338

Rickard, W. (1998). Oral history – 'more dangerous than therapy'?:
Interviewees' reflections on recording traumatic or taboo issues. *Oral
History, 26*(2), 34–48. https://www.jstor.org/stable/40179520

Rodéhn, C. (2020). The happy teacher: A critical exploration of the joys
of object-based learning and teaching in higher education. In T. Kador &
H. Chatterjee (Eds.), *Object-based learning and well-being* (pp.140–156).
London: Routledge.

Romein, C. A., Kemman, M. Birkholz, J. M., Baker, J., De Gruijter, M.,
Meroño-Peñuela, A., ... Scagliola, S. (2020). State of the field: Digital
history. *History, 105*(365), 291–312. http://dx.doi.org/10.1111/
1468-229X.12969

Rosenberg, F., Parsa, A., Humble, L., & McGee, C. (2009). *Meet me:
Making art accessible to people with dementia*. New York, NY: Museum
of Modern Art, New York.

Rosenzweig, R., & Thelen, D. (2012). The presence of the past: Popular
uses of history in American life. In P. Ashton & H. Kean (Eds.), *Public
history and heritage today: People and their pasts* (pp. 30–55). London:
Palgrave Macmillan.

Rosner, D., & Markowitz, G. (2019). An enormous victory for public
health in California: Industries are responsible for cleaning up the

environments they polluted. *American Journal of Public Health*, 109(2), 211–212. https://doi.org/10.2105/ajph.2018.304887

Rothman, D. J. (2003). Serving clio and client: The historian as expert witness. *Bulletin of the History of Medicine*, 77(1), 25–44. https://doi.org/10.1353/bhm.2003.0035

Russell, C., Kohe, G. Z., Brooker, D., & Evans, S. (2019). Sporting identity, memory, and people with dementia: Opportunities, challenges, and potential for oral history. *The International Journal of the History of Sport*, 36(13–14), 1157–1179. https://doi.org/10.1080/09523367.2019.1703690

Saavedra, J., Español, A., Arias-Sánchez, S., & Calderón-Garcia, M. (2017). *Creative practices for improving health and social inclusion.* Seville: University of Seville Press.

Scally, G., & Womack, J. (2004). The importance of the past in public health. *Journal of Epidemiology and Community Health*, 58(9), 751–755. https://doi.org/10.1136/jech.2003.014340

Sedikides, C., & Wildschut, T. (2016). Past forward: Nostalgia as a motivational force. *Trends in Cognitive Sciences*, 20(5), 319–321. https://doi.org/10.1016/j.tics.2016.01.008

Sheard, S. (2008). History *in* health and health services: Exploring the possibilities. *Journal of Epidemiology & Community Health*, 62(8), 740–744. https://doi.org/10.1136/jech.2007.063412

Sheard, S. (2018). History matters: The critical contribution of historical analysis to contemporary health policy and health care. *Health Care Analysis*, 26(2), 140–154. https://doi.org/10.1007/s10728-017-0348-4

Simpson, J. M., Checkland, K., Snow, S. J., Voorhees, J., Rothwell, K., & Esmail, A. (2018). Adding the past to the policy mix: An historical approach to the issue of access to general practice in England. *Contemporary British History*, 32(2), 276–299. https://doi.org/10.1080/13619462.2017.1401474

Smith, C., Copley, V., Lower, K., Kotaba, A., & Jackson, G. (2022). Using archaeology to strengthen Indigenous social, emotional, and economic wellbeing. In P. Everill & K. Burnell (Eds.), *Archaeology, heritage, and wellbeing* (pp. 119–144). London: Routledge.

Snow, C. P. (1959). *The two cultures and the scientific revolution.* Cambridge: Cambridge University Press.

Thompson, J., Brown, Z., Baker, K., Naisby, J., Mitchell, S., Dodds, C., ... Collins, T. (2020). Development of the 'Museum Health and Social Care Service' to promote the use of arts and cultural activities by health and social care professionals caring for older people. *Educational Gerontology, 46*(8), 452–460. https://doi.org/10.1080/03601277.2020. 1770469

Thompson, P. with Bornat, J. (2017, first published 1978). *The voice of the past: Oral history.* Oxford: Oxford University Press.

Thomson, A. (2015). *Anzac Memories* revisited: Trauma, memory and oral history. *Oral History Review, 42*(1), 1–29. https://doi.org/10.1093/ ohr/ohv010. This provides further reflections on his book: Thompson, A. (1994). *Anzac memories: Living with the legend.* Oxford: Oxford University Press.

Thomson, L. J., & Chatterjee, H. J. (2015). Measuring the impact of museum activities on well-being: Developing the museum well-being measures toolkit. *Museum Management and Curatorship, 30*(1), 44–62. https://doi.org/10.1080/09647775.2015.1008390

Tomes, N. (1991). Oral history in the history of medicine. *The Journal of American History, 78*(2), 607–617. https://doi.org/10.2307/2079538

Tosh, J. (2008). *Why history matters.* London: Palgrave Macmillan.

Tosh, J. (2015, first published 1984). *The pursuit of history: Aims, methods, and new directions in the study of history.* London: Routledge.

Vyas, D. A., Eisenstein, L. G., & Jones, D. S., (2020). Hidden in plain sight—Reconsidering the use of race correction in clinical algorithm. *The New England Journal of Medicine, 383*, 874–882. https://doi. org/10.1056/NEJMms2004740

Wakefield, D. (2007). The future of medical museums: Threatened but not extinct. *Medical Journal of Australia, 187*(7), 380-381. https://doi.org/ 10.5694/j.1326-5377.2007.tb01304.x

Whitehouse, S. (2019). A lead-abatement judgment driven by science, history, and the law. *American Journal of Public Health, 109*(4), 544. https://doi.org/10.2105/ajph.2019.304983

Wilson, M. (2022). *Arts for health: Storytelling*. Bingley: Emerald Books.

Winslow, M., Hitchlock, K., & Noble, B. (2009). Recording lives: The benefits of an oral history service. *European Journal of Palliative Care*, *16*(3), 128–130. Retrieved from https://pascal-francis.inist.fr/vibad/index. php?action=getRecordDetail&idt=21730927

Winslow, M., & Smith, G. (2010). Ethical challenges in the oral history of medicine. In D. Ritchie (Ed.), *The Oxford handbook of oral history* (pp. 372–392). Oxford: Oxford University Press.

Woods, A. (2001, February 28). Kill or cure? *The Guardian*. Retrieved from https://www.theguardian.com/society/2001/feb/28/ guardiansocietysupplement4

INDEX

Printed in the USA
CPSIA information can be obtained
at www.ICGtesting.com
JSHW050542230923
48989JS00001B/1